A Step Above

50 Easy DIY Disinfectant Spray's

BY

Alice R. Groner

License Notes

No part of this Book can be reproduced in any form or by any means including print, electronic, scanning or photocopying unless prior permission is granted by the author.

All ideas, suggestions and guidelines mentioned here are written for informative purposes. While the author has taken every possible step to ensure accuracy, all readers are advised to follow information at their own risk. The author cannot be held responsible for personal and/or commercial damages in case of misinterpreting and misunderstanding any part of this Book

Table of Contents

Introduction 7

Tips 9

Basic Disinfecting Spray (DIY LYSOL SPRAY) 10

DIY Disinfecting Wipes with Isopropyl Alcohol 11

DIY Disinfecting Wipes with Ethanol Alcohol 13

Straight 70% Alcohol Spray 15

Disinfecting Thyme 16

Disinfecting Lemon Thyme Bathroom and Kitchen Disinfectant 18

Sunny Day Disinfectant Spray 20

Clean Thyme Disinfecting Spray 22

Lavender Thyme Bedroom Disinfectant 24

Lemon & Lavender Disinfecting Spray 26

Faux Lysol Wipes with Tea Tree Oil 28

15 oz. Lemon Thyme Disinfecting Spray 30

15 oz Lemon & Lavender Appliance Disinfectant 32

Minty Disinfectant Spray 34

X-tra Minty Disinfectant 36

Sage Disinfecting Spray 38

Eucalyptus Blu Disinfecting Spray 40

Lavender & Eucalyptus Blu Disinfecting Spray 42

Lavender & Sage Disinfecting Spray 44

Eucalyptus & Rose Disinfecting Spray for High Traffic Areas 46

Lemon-Sage Disinfecting Spray 48

Lemon DIY Disinfecting Wipes with Isopropyl Alcohol 50

Lemon DIY Disinfecting Wipes with Ethanol Alcohol 52

Lemon Thyme Disinfecting Wipes with Isopropyl Alcohol 54

Lemon-Thyme Disinfecting Car Wipes with Ethanol Alcohol 56

Lemon Rose Power Wipes with Isopropyl Alcohol 58

DIY Multi-Purpose Disinfecting Wipes with Ethanol Alcohol 60

DIY Easy Extra Strength Disinfecting Wipes 62

Extra Strength Disinfecting Wipes with Ethanol Alcohol 64

Easy DIY All-Purpose Cleaner with Vodka 66

Easy DIY All-Purpose Cleaner Wipes with Vodka 67

DIY Kitchen All-Purpose Cleaner Wipes with Vodka 69

DIY Disinfectant Spray for Granite Counters 71

DIY Disinfectant Wipes for Granite Counters 73

L & L Disinfectant Wipes for Granite Counters 75

Grapefruit Disinfectant Wipes for Granite Counters 77

Orange-Sage Disinfectant Spray for Granite Counters 79

Easy Bleach Disinfectant 81

Clorox Recommended Disinfect Spray 83

DIY Bleach Wipes 84

Disinfecting Glass Cleaner 86

Homemade Anti-Bacterial Wipes 88

Lemon & Coconut Disinfecting Wipes 90

Lavender and Eucalyptus Disinfecting Wipes 92

Cinna-mon Wipes 94

Citrus Disinfecting Wipes 96

Grapefruit & Lavender Disinfecting Spray 98

Lemon Rose Disinfecting Wipes 100

Eucalyptus Blu All-Purpose Cleaner Wipes with Vodka 102

Heavy Duty Shop Wipes with Vodka 104

Black Rose Disinfecting Wipes.. 106

White Rose Wipes with Vodka 108

Author's Afterthoughts.. 110

Introduction

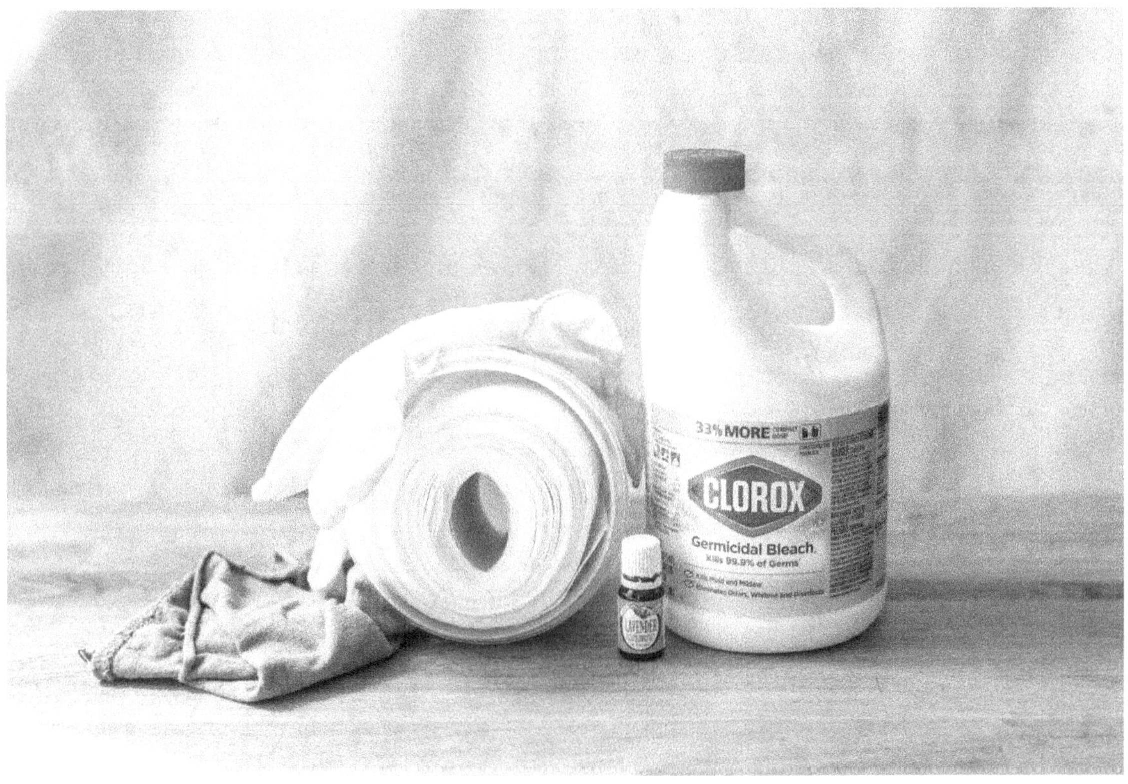

Do you know the difference between sanitizing and disinfecting? The words are used interchangeably, but they are not the same. A disinfectant offers a higher level of germ removal. Sanitizing is comparable to your basic hand sanitizer: it removes 60-80 percent of germs, whereas, disinfecting removes 85%-97%. CDC guidelines recommend disinfectant, in 1 of 3 strengths, due to its prolonged ability to greatly reduce or eliminate germs and pathogens.

A Step Above: 50 Easy DIY Disinfectant Spray's gives you 50 easy DIY disinfectant recipes. All fall within CDC guidelines for 1 of 3 strengths disinfectant sprays and wipes with easy to find, eco-friendly ingredients, such as vinegar, peroxide, alcohol. Mixed with fresh, bright colors and scents from your favorite essential oils.

A Step Above: 50 Easy DIY Disinfectant Spray's has a wipe or spray for all your household DIY disinfectant needs!

A chemical smell doesn't always equal clean. Sometimes it means being sick and another unproductive day. Don't give up any more of your life, time, or energy. A Step Above: 50 Easy DIY Disinfectant Spray's makes the disinfecting process quick, easy, and harmless. Natural ingredient for strong disinfecting for all your household needs.

Tips

1.) Isopropyl alcohol can be purchased at stores and is frequently found in hand sanitizer.

2.) Ethanol alcohol is drunk.

3.) According to certain studies, isopropyl alcohol is better for eliminating bacteria and ethanol is better for eliminating the virus.

4.) Only use vodka in a disinfectant spray or wipe if it is at least 130 proof and don't use any water.

5.) Alcohol less than 70% is ineffective against viruses.

6.) Bleach lessens in strength a little every day once removed from its original container. Never make more than a few days' worths at a time.

7.) Prolonged exposure to sunlight will weaken bleach. Keep stored in a cabinet or similar dark space.

8.) Never mix bleach with ammonia or vinegar.

Basic Disinfecting Spray (DIY LYSOL SPRAY)

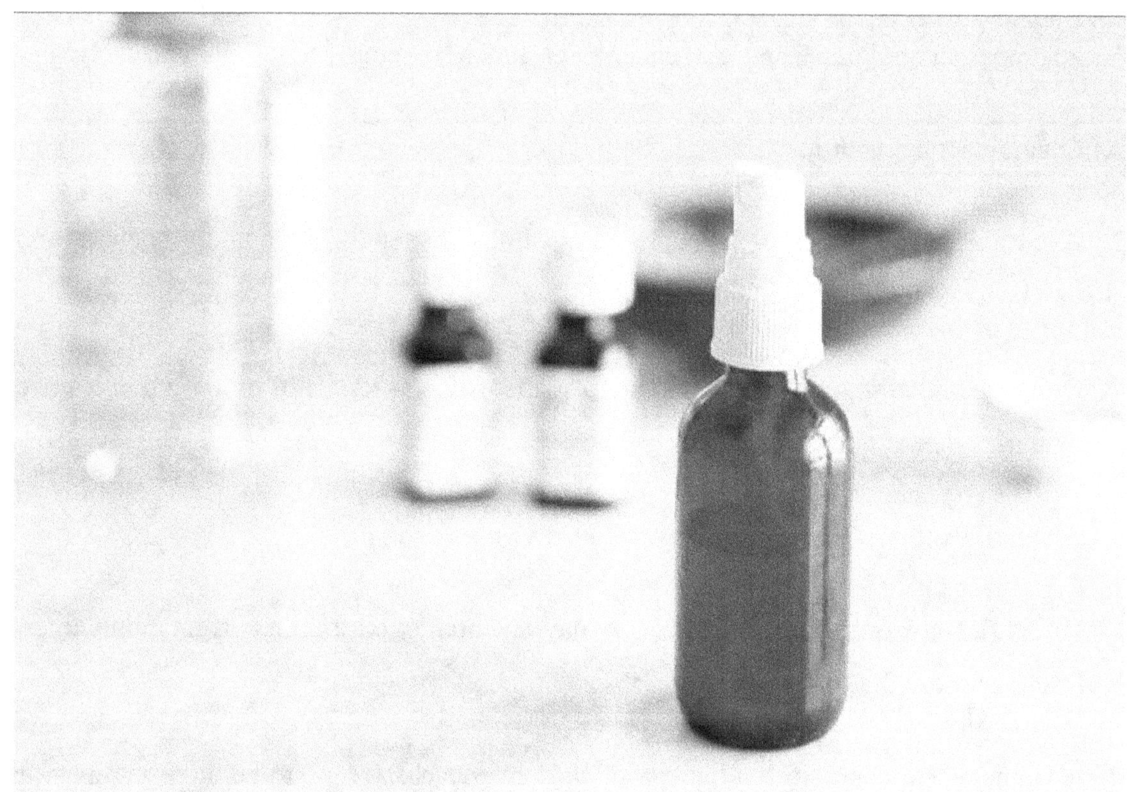

Great for high touch surfaces; makes approx. 13-16 oz.

Ingredients:

- 3 oz sterile water
- 10 oz alcohol
- ¼-1/3 tsp peroxide

Instructions:

In a spray bottle mix together water, alcohol, peroxide.

DIY Disinfecting Wipes with Isopropyl Alcohol

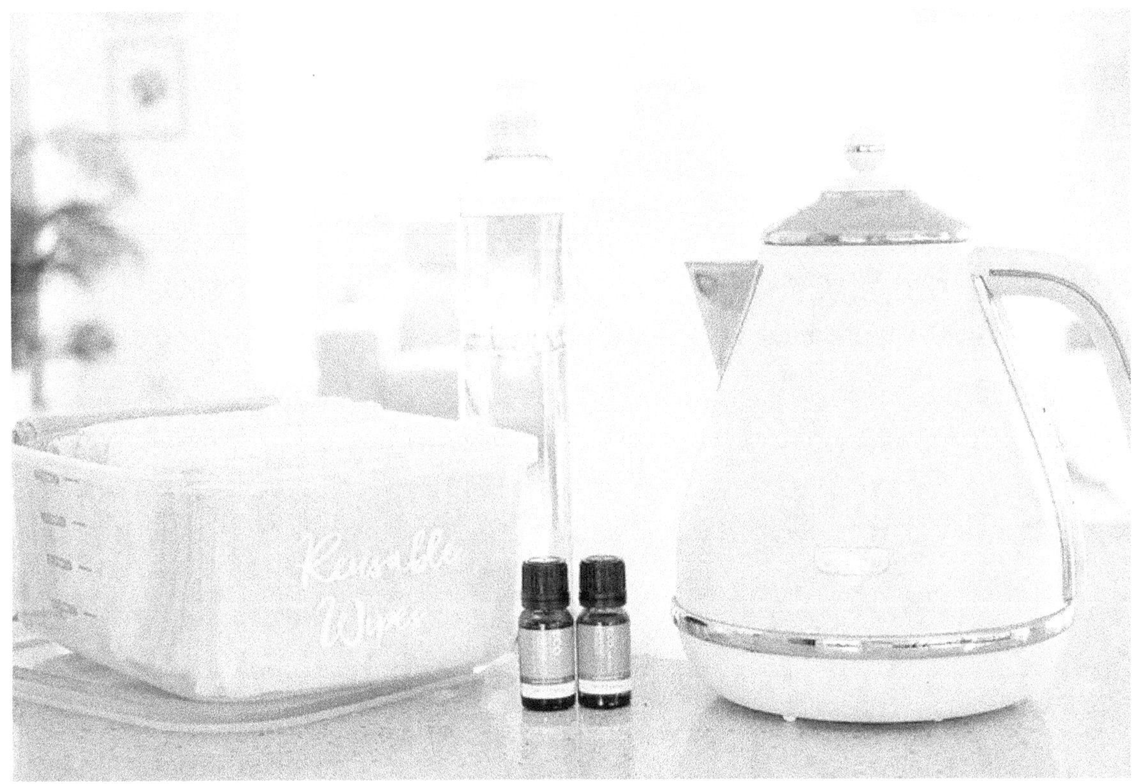

Cut paper-towels in half and put them in a baby wipe container! Makes approx. 150-180 wipes.

Ingredients:

- 16-18 oz 91-99% isopropyl alcohol
- 3-5 oz sterile water
- 1 ½ tsp peroxide

Instructions:

Mix together alcohol, water, peroxide. Submerge papers towels into mixture. Let drain and stick inside a jar or container.

DIY Disinfecting Wipes with Ethanol Alcohol

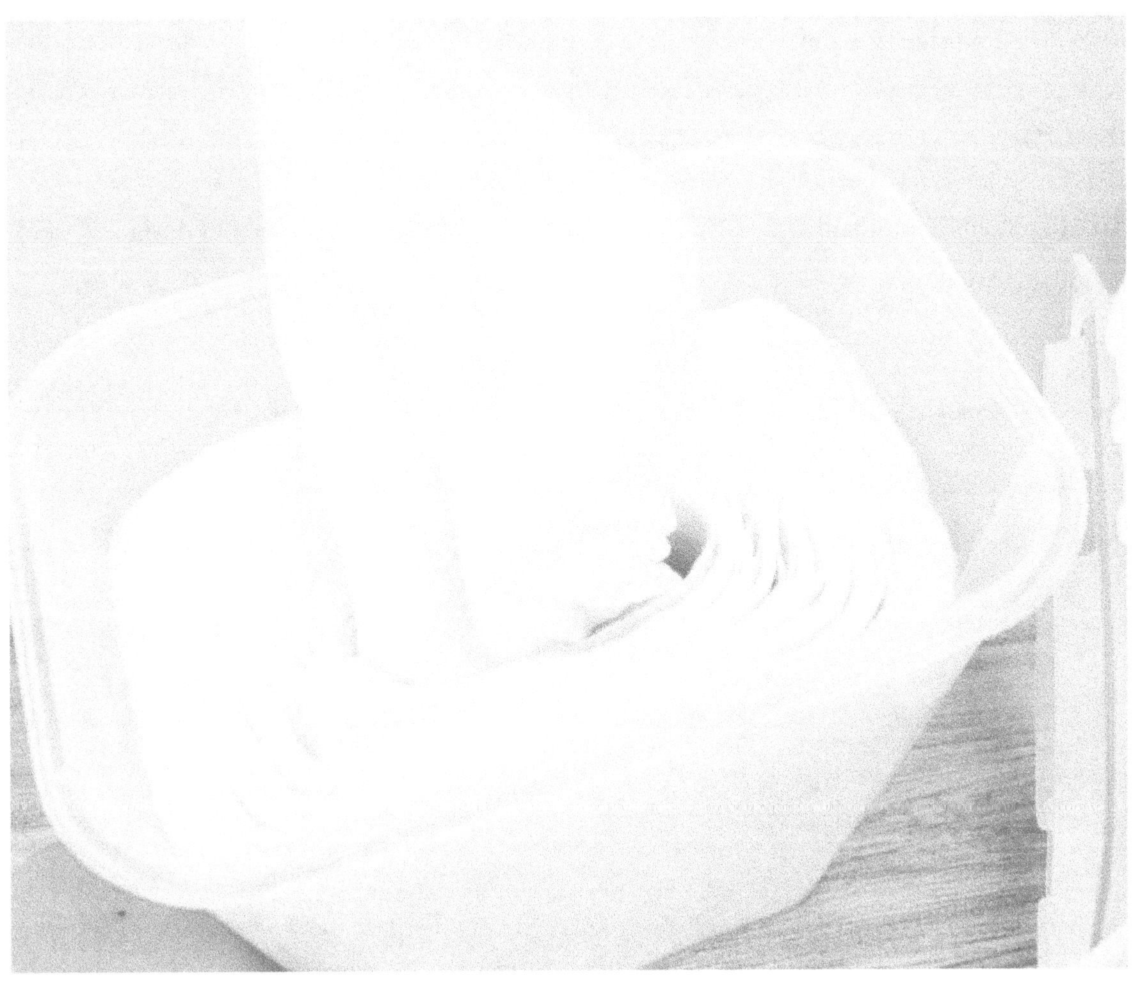

Good for cell phones and keyboards. Makes approx. 150-180 wipes.

Ingredients:

- 16-18 oz ethanol alcohol
- 1-2 oz sterile water

Instructions:

Mix together alcohol and water. Submerge papers towels into mixture. Let drain and stick inside a jar or container.

Straight 70% Alcohol Spray

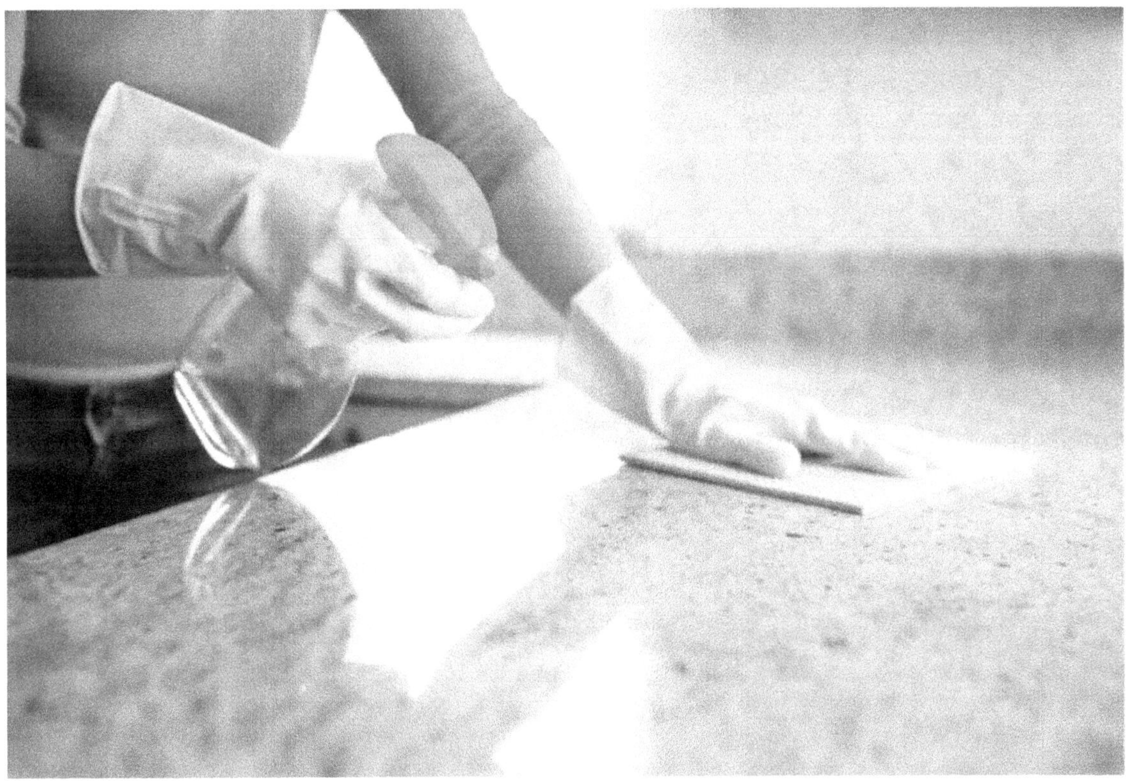

70% or higher isopropyl alcohol will eliminate virus! Makes approx. 14-18 oz.

Ingredients:

- 14-18 oz

Instructions:

Pour into spray bottle and disinfect kitchens and bathrooms!

Disinfecting Thyme

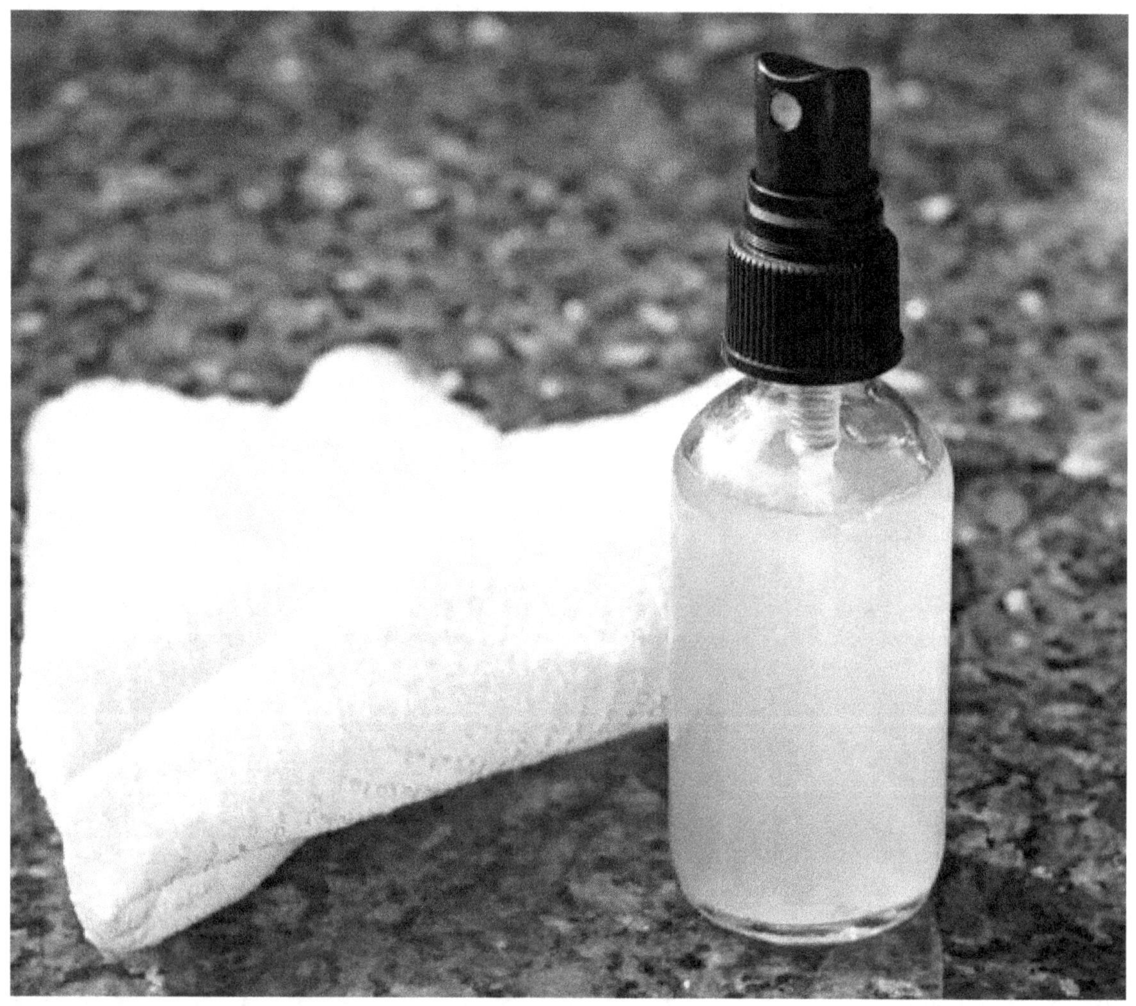

Great smelling! Makes 6-8 oz.

Ingredients:

- 7-8 oz. sterile water
- 20-30 drops thyme essential oil
- ½-1 tsp 70 % alcohol

Instructions:

In spray bottle mix together water, thyme, and alcohol.

Disinfecting Lemon Thyme Bathroom and Kitchen Disinfectant

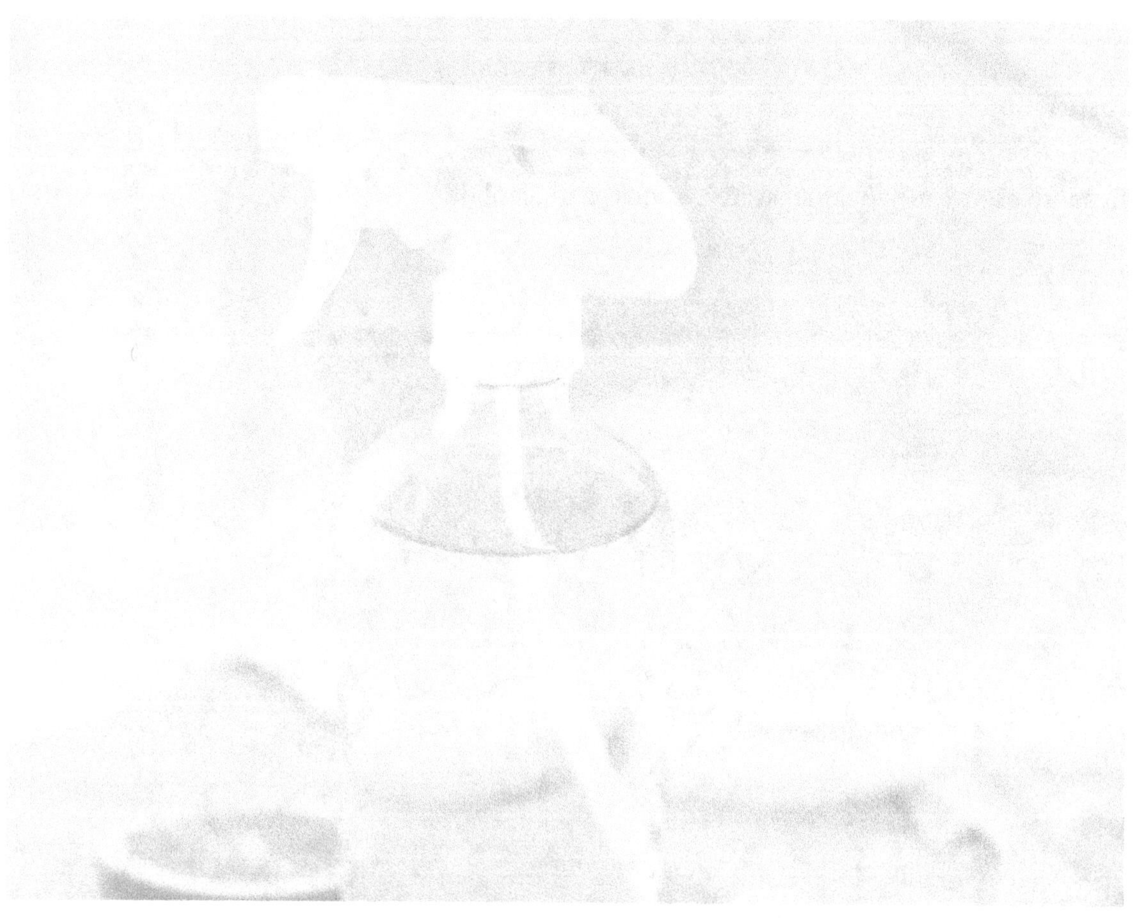

Sub 5-8 drops of tea tree oil for the thyme! Makes 6-8 oz.

Ingredients:

- 7-8 oz. sterile water
- 15 drops lemon essential oil
- 20-30 drops thyme essential oil
- ½-1 tsp 70 % alcohol

Instructions:

In spray bottle mix together water, lemon, thyme, and alcohol.

Sunny Day Disinfectant Spray

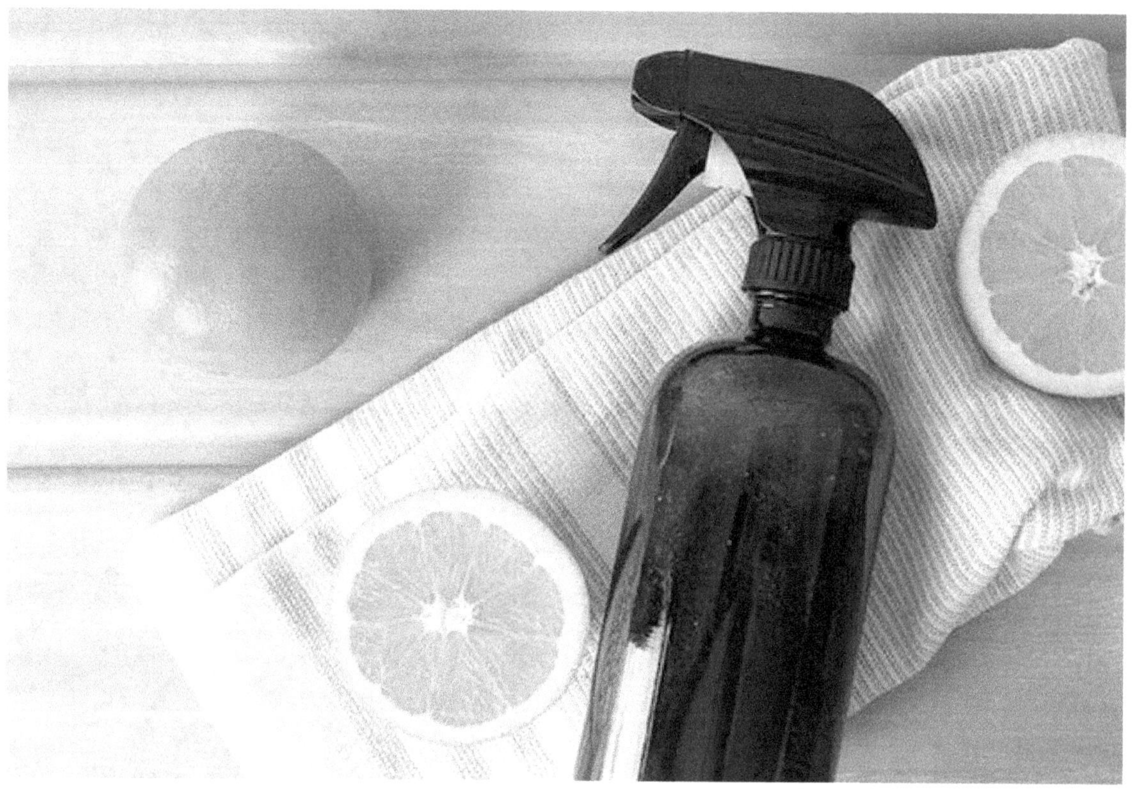

Fresh, invigorating, and germ eliminating! Makes 6-8 oz.

Ingredients:

- 7-8 oz. sterile water
- 15 drops orange essential oil
- 25-30 drops thyme essential oil
- ½-1 tsp isopropyl 70 % alcohol

Instructions:

In spray bottle mix together water, orange, thyme, and alcohol.

Clean Thyme Disinfecting Spray

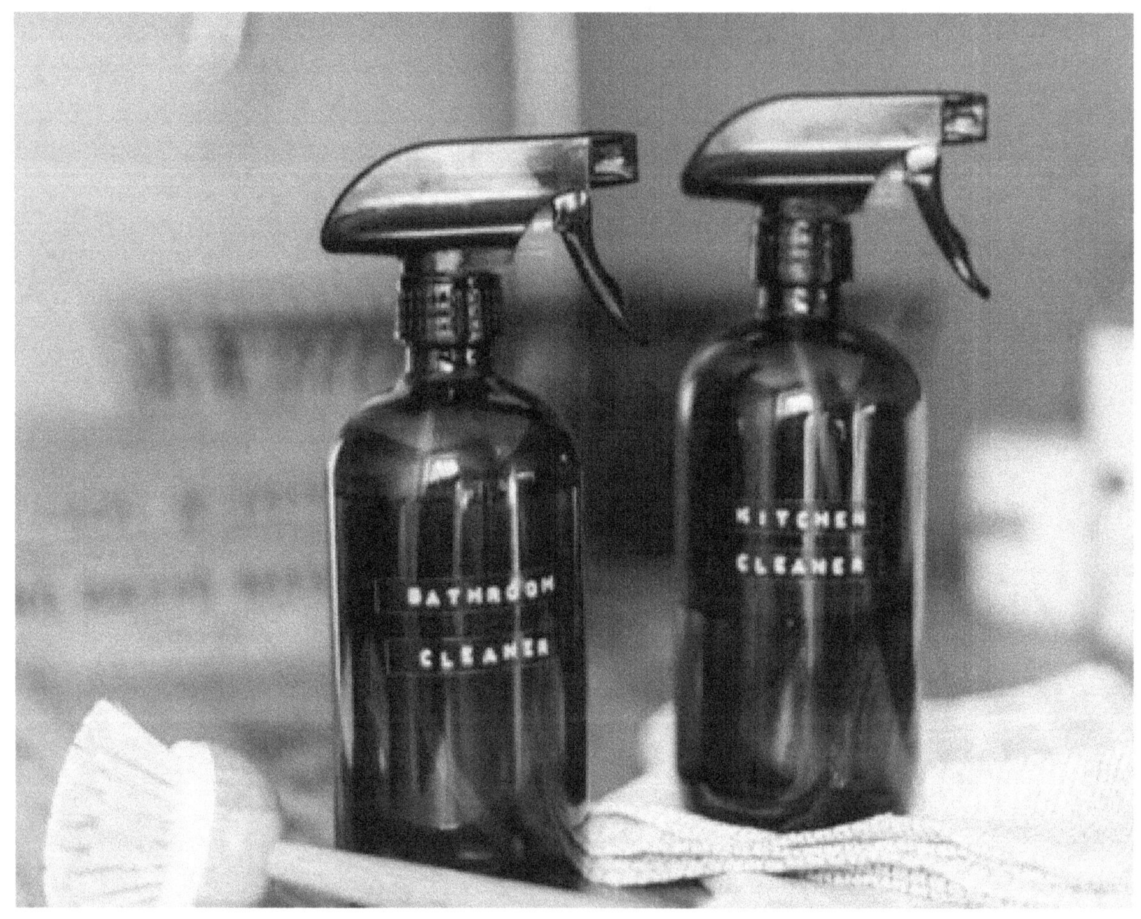

Great for bedrooms and dens! Makes 6-8 oz.

Ingredients:

- 7-8 oz. sterile water
- 20 drops of grapefruit oil
- 20-30 drops thyme essential oil
- ½-1 tsp 70 % isopropyl alcohol

Instructions:

In spray bottle mix together water, grapefruit and thyme, and alcohol.

Lavender Thyme Bedroom Disinfectant

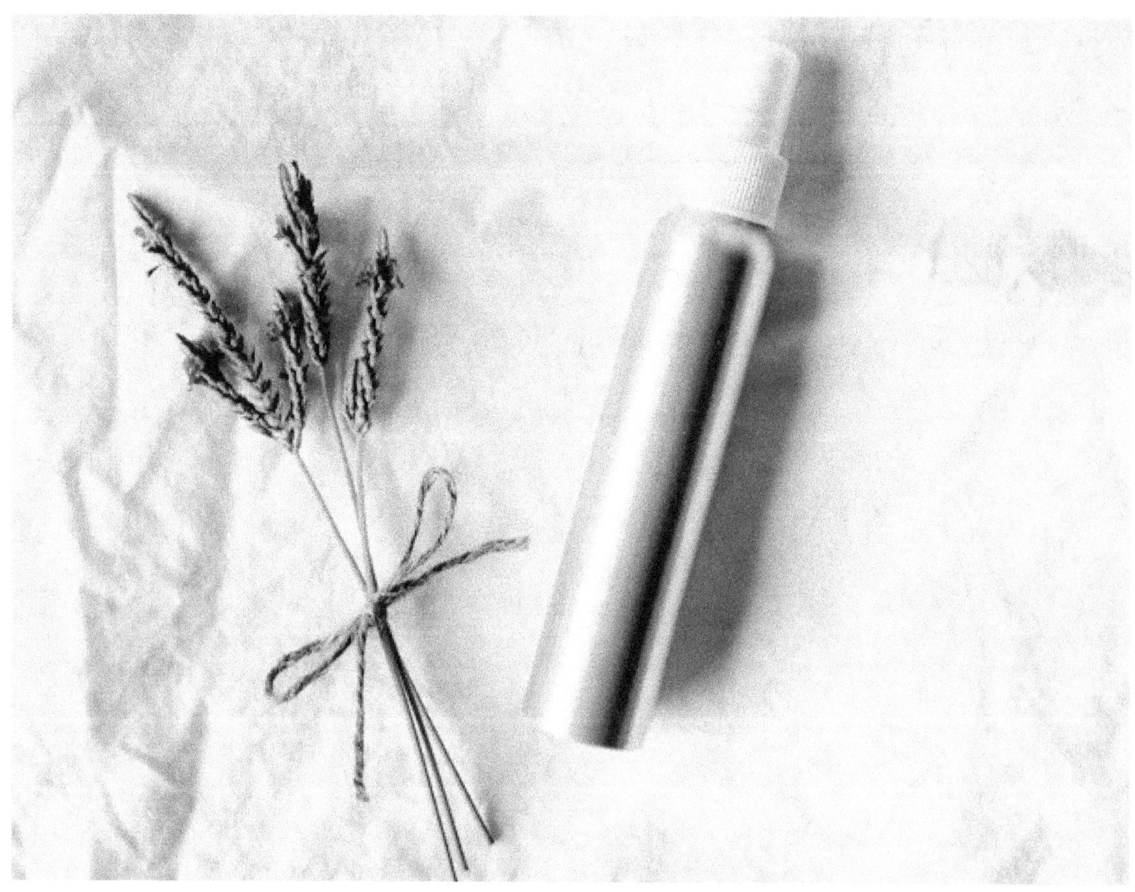

Lavender is great for relaxing! Makes 6-8 oz.

Ingredients:

- 7-8 oz. sterile water
- 20-30 drops thyme essential oil
- ½-1 tsp 70 % alcohol

Instructions:

In spray bottle mix together water, thyme, and alcohol.

Lemon & Lavender Disinfecting Spray

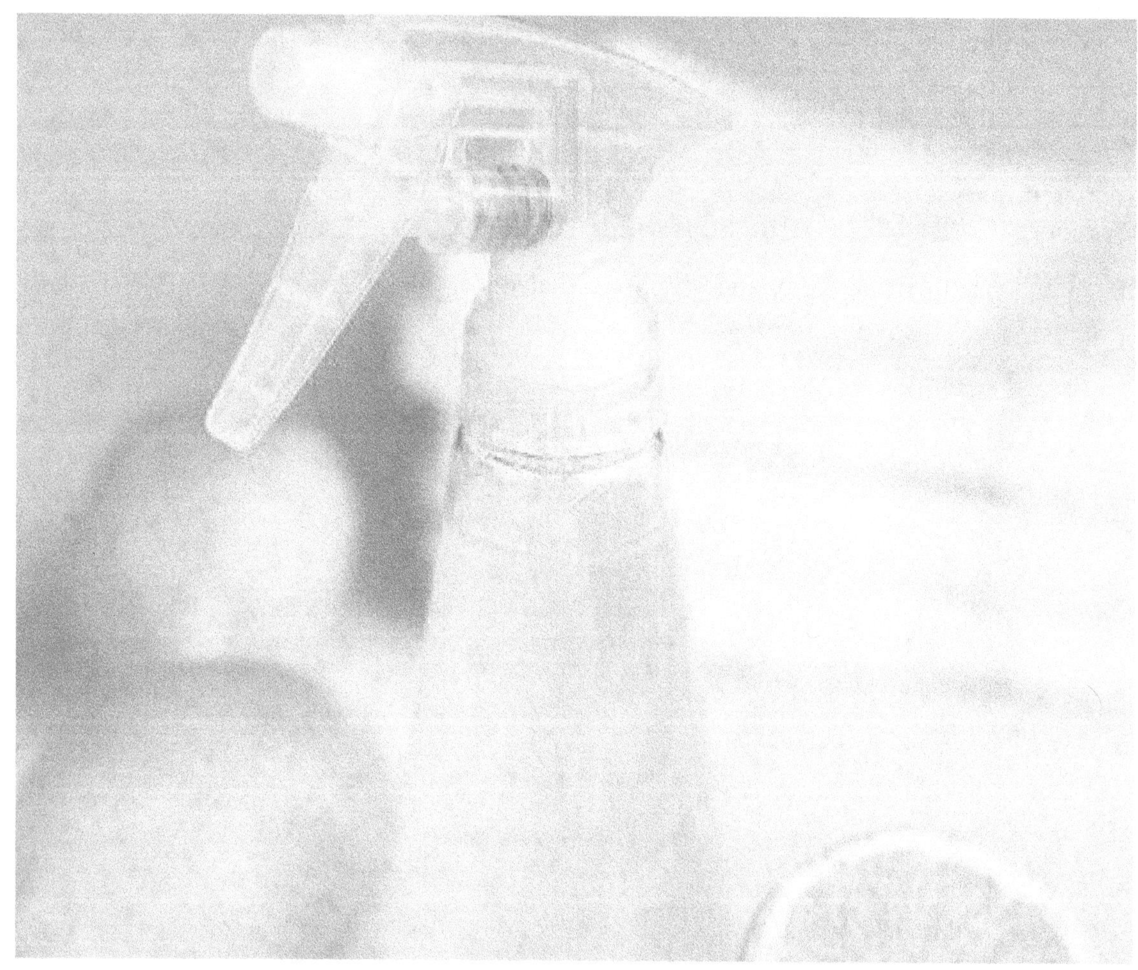

Keep a bottle in the car! Makes 6-8 oz.

Ingredients:

- 7-8 oz. sterile water
- 30 drops lemon essential oil
- 20 drops lavender essential oil
- ½-1 tsp 70 % alcohol

Instructions:

In spray bottle mix together water, lemon & lavender, and alcohol.

Faux Lysol Wipes with Tea Tree Oil

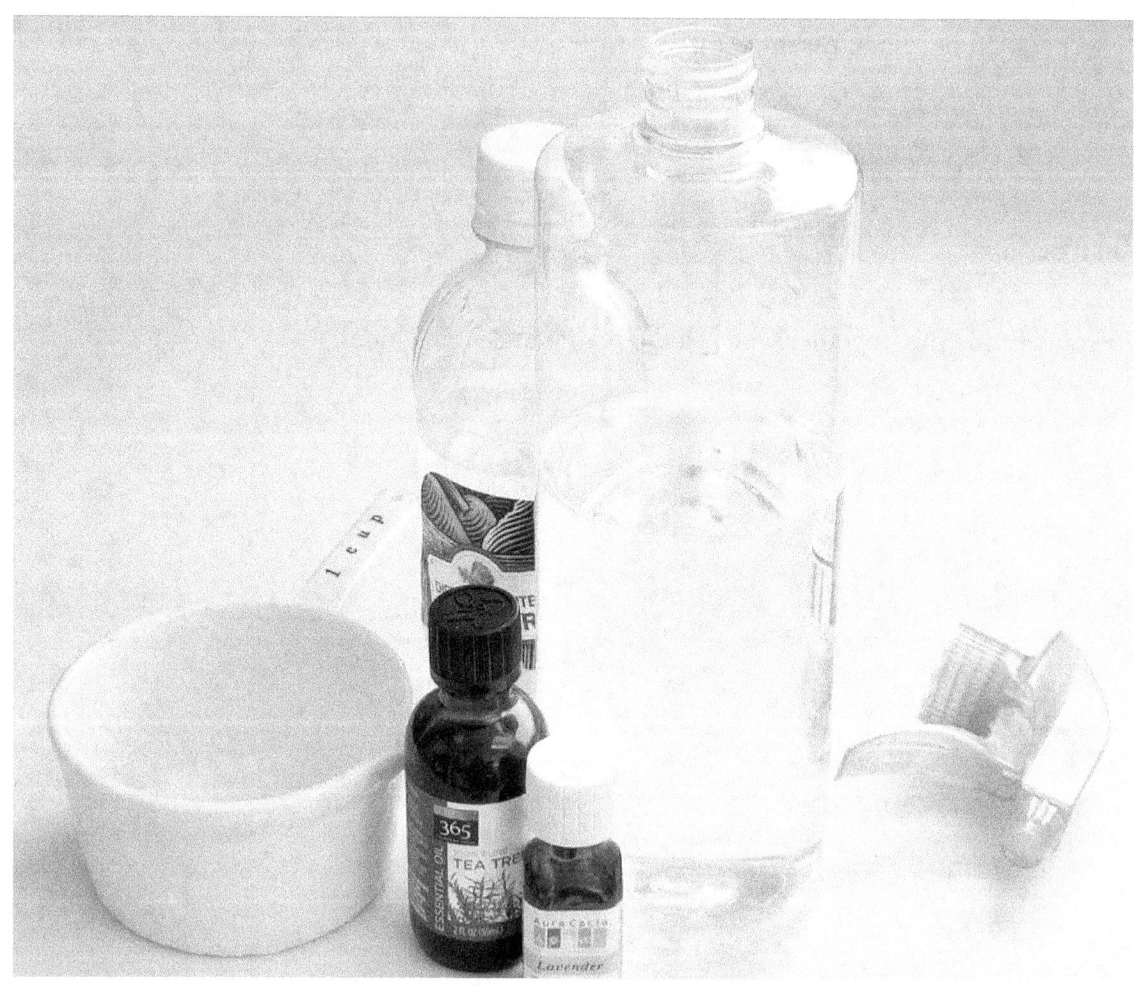

Great for high touch surfaces; makes approx. 13-16 oz.

Ingredients:

- 3 oz sterile water
- 10 oz alcohol
- ¼-1/3 tsp peroxide
- 5 drops of tea tree oil

Instructions:

In a spray bottle mix together water, alcohol, peroxide, tea tree oil.

15 oz. Lemon Thyme Disinfecting Spray

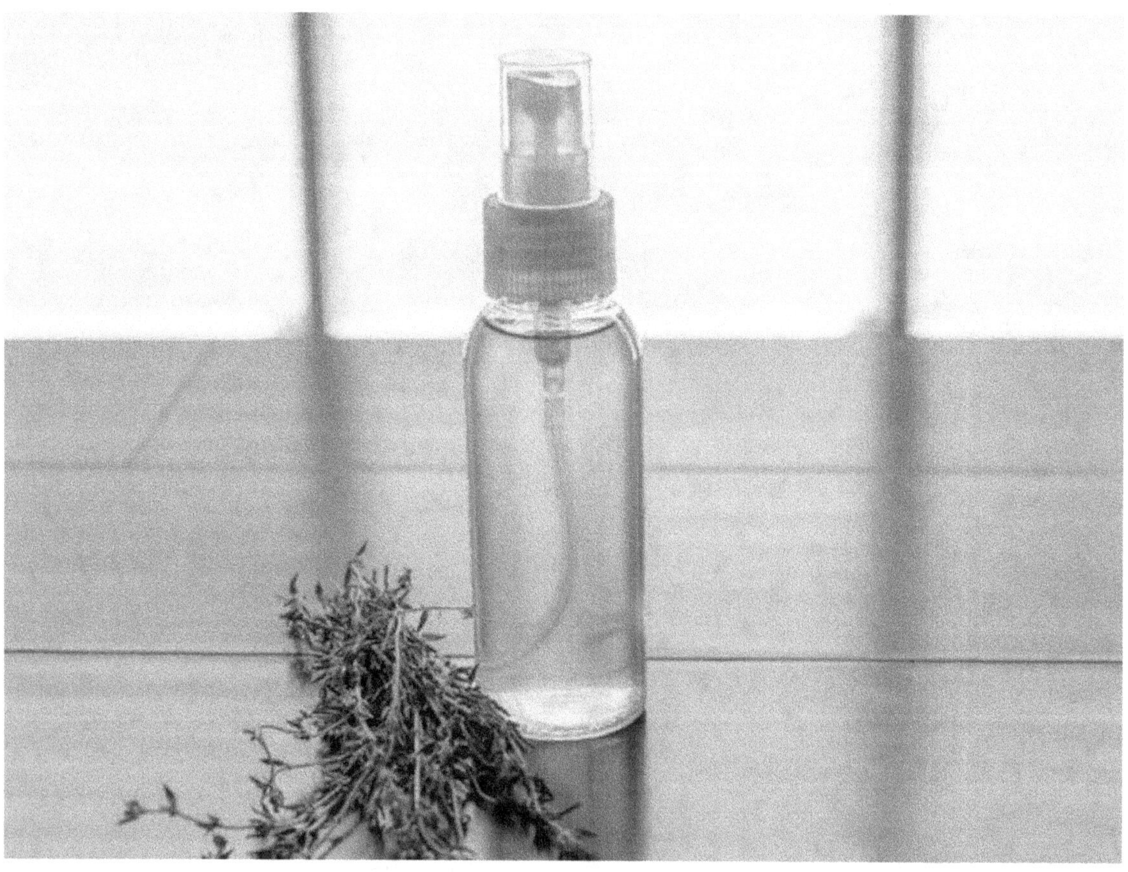

Great for porous surfaces; makes 15 oz.

Ingredients:

- 3 oz sterile water
- 10-12 oz alcohol
- ¼-1/3 tsp peroxide
- 30 drops of lemon essential oil
- 20 drops thyme essential oil

Instructions:

In a spray bottle mix together water, alcohol, peroxide, lemon, thyme.

15 oz Lemon & Lavender Appliance Disinfectant

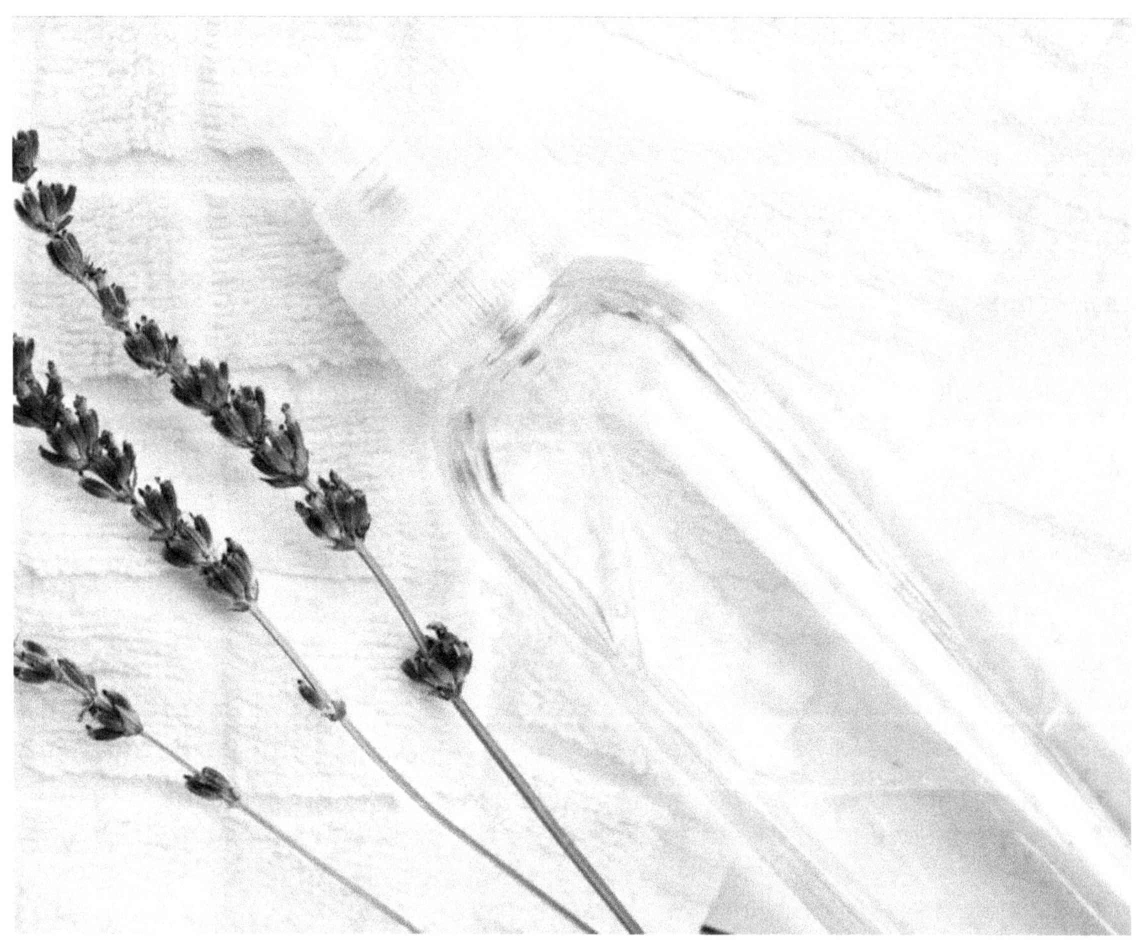

Great for living rooms, offices, and dens; makes 15 oz.

Ingredients:

- 3 oz sterile water
- 10-12 oz alcohol
- ¼-1/3 tsp peroxide
- 30 drops of lemon essential oil
- 18-22 drops lavender essential oil

Instructions:

In a spray bottle mix together water, alcohol, peroxide, lemon & lavender.

Minty Disinfectant Spray

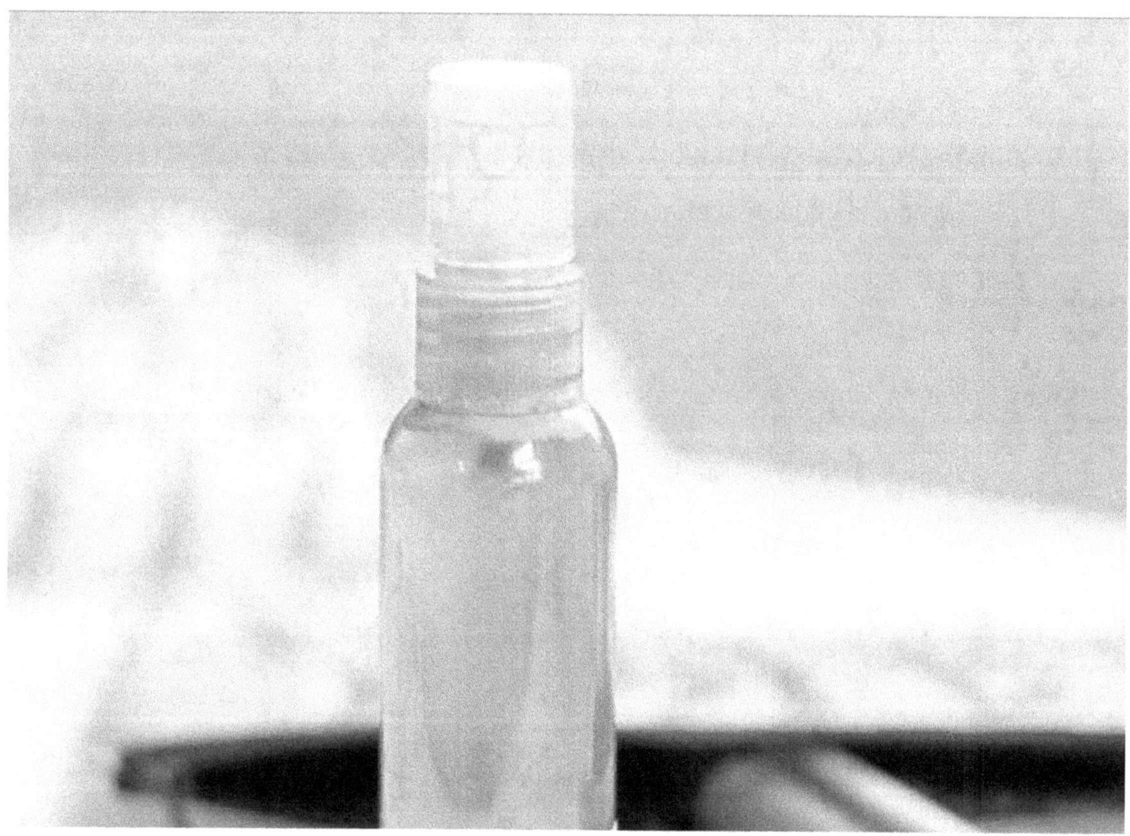

Smells great; makes approx. 13-16 oz.

Ingredients:

- 3 oz sterile water
- 10 oz alcohol
- ¼-1/3 tsp peroxide
- 20-25 drops of peppermint essential oil
- 5-10 drops of thyme essential oil

Instructions:

In a spray bottle mix together water, alcohol, peroxide, peppermint & thyme.

X-tra Minty Disinfectant

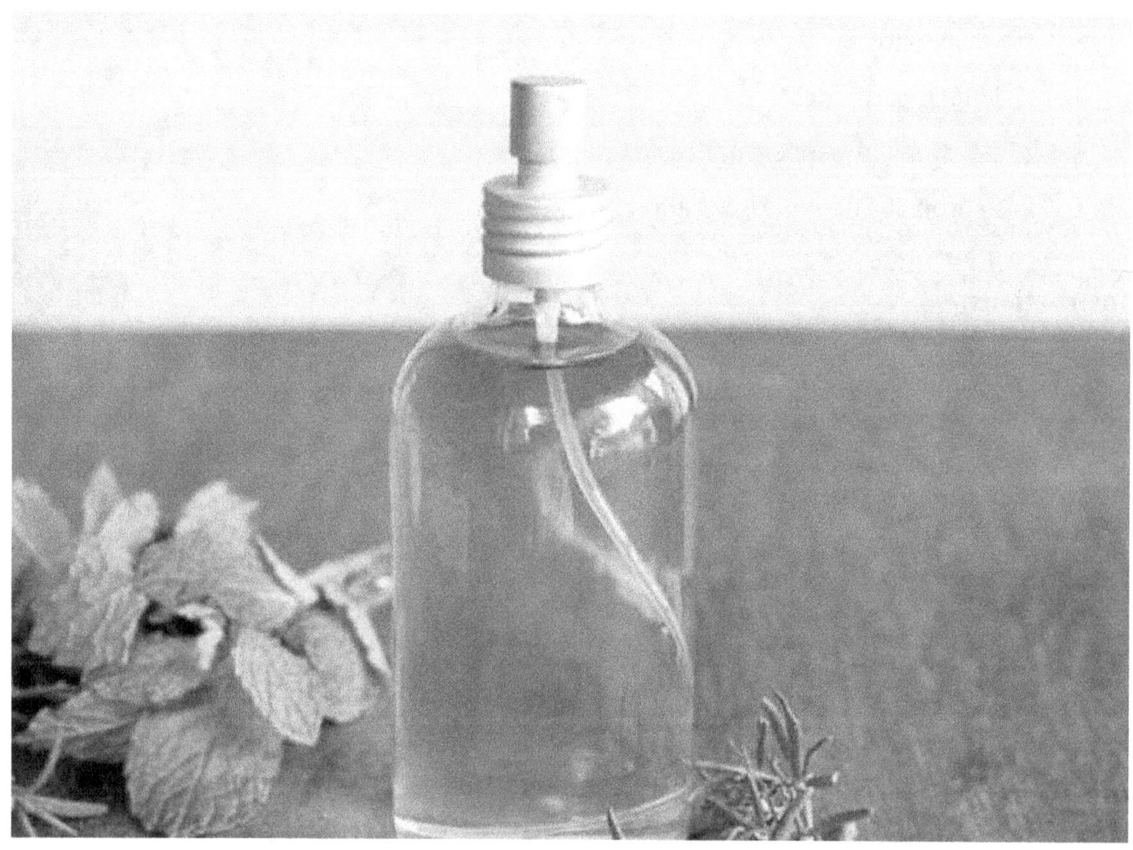

Great for bedrooms and utility rooms; makes approx. 13-16 oz.

Ingredients:

- 3 oz sterile water
- 10 oz alcohol
- ¼-1/3 tsp peroxide
- 20 drops peppermint essential oil
- 5-7 drops tea tree essential oil

Instructions:

In a spray bottle mix together water, alcohol, peroxide, peppermint and tea tree oils.

Sage Disinfecting Spray

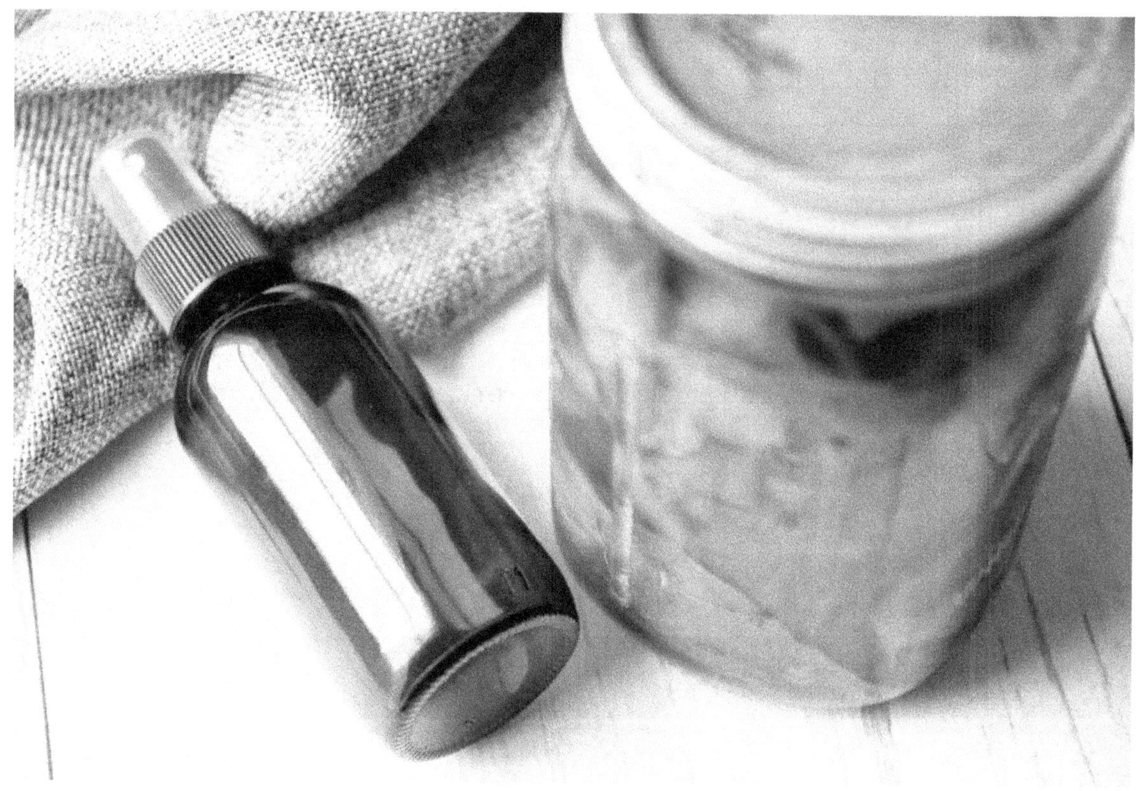

Great for garages, cars, and tools; makes approx. 13-16 oz.

Ingredients:

- 3 oz sterile water
- 10 oz alcohol
- ¼-1/3 tsp peroxide
- 20-30 drops sage essential oil
- 3-5 drops thyme or tea tree oil
- 5-8 drops sage food coloring

Instructions:

In a spray bottle mix together water, alcohol, peroxide, sage & thyme or tea tree oil, green food coloring.

Eucalyptus Blu Disinfecting Spray

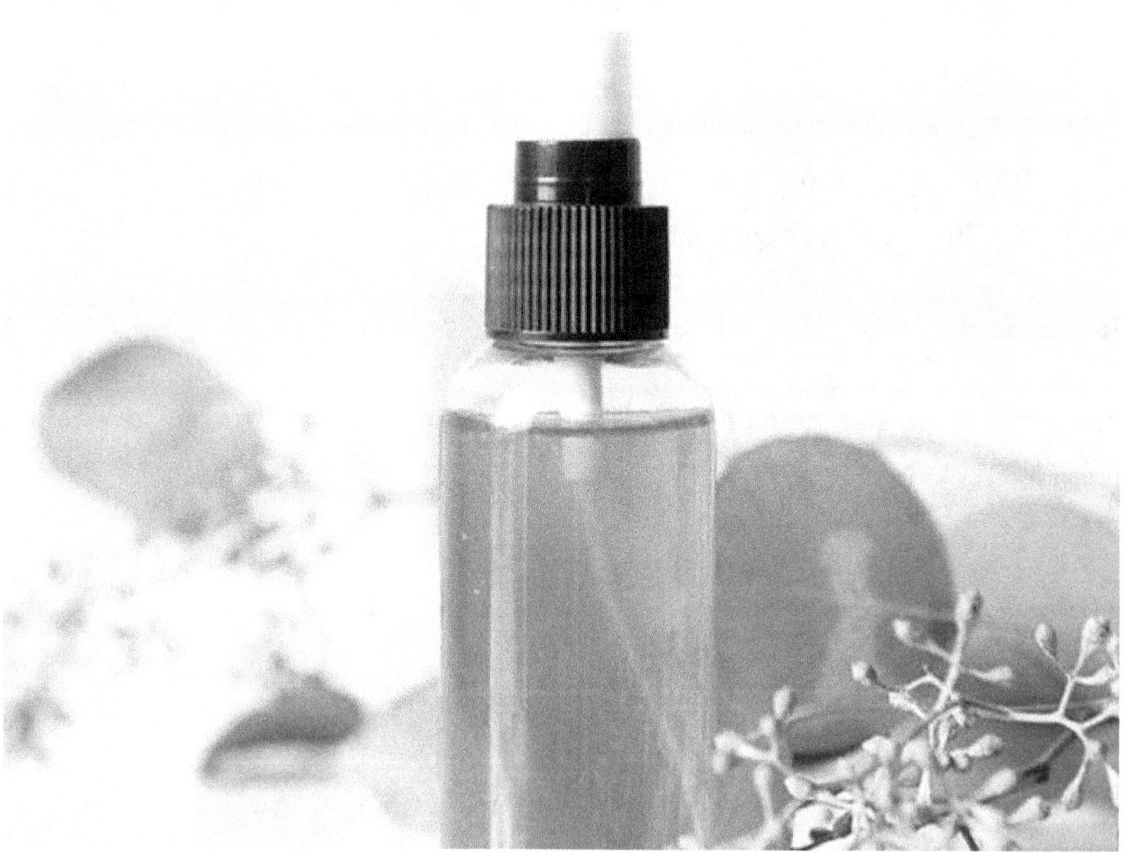

Great for garages; makes approx. 13-16 oz.

Ingredients:

- 3 oz sterile water

- 10 oz alcohol

- ¼-1/3 tsp peroxide

- 20-30 drops eucalyptus essential oil

• 5-8 drops blue food coloring

Instructions:

In a spray bottle mix together water, alcohol, peroxide, eucalyptus oil, blue food coloring.

Lavender & Eucalyptus Blu Disinfecting Spray

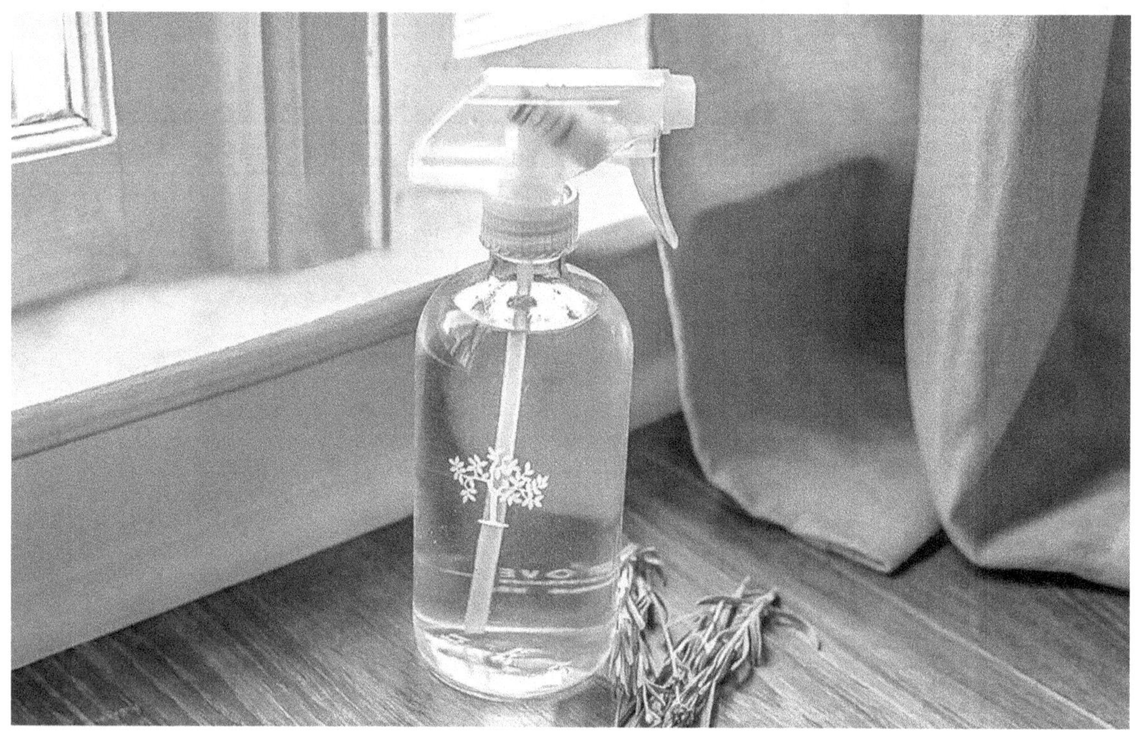

Great for garages, sheds, and cleaning tools; makes approx. 13-16 oz.

Ingredients:

- 3 oz sterile water
- 10 oz alcohol
- ¼-1/3 tsp peroxide
- 20 drops eucalyptus essential oil
- 10-12 drops lavender essential oil
- 5-8 drops blue food coloring

Instructions:

In a spray bottle mix together water, alcohol, peroxide, eucalyptus & lavender oils, blue food coloring.

Lavender & Sage Disinfecting Spray

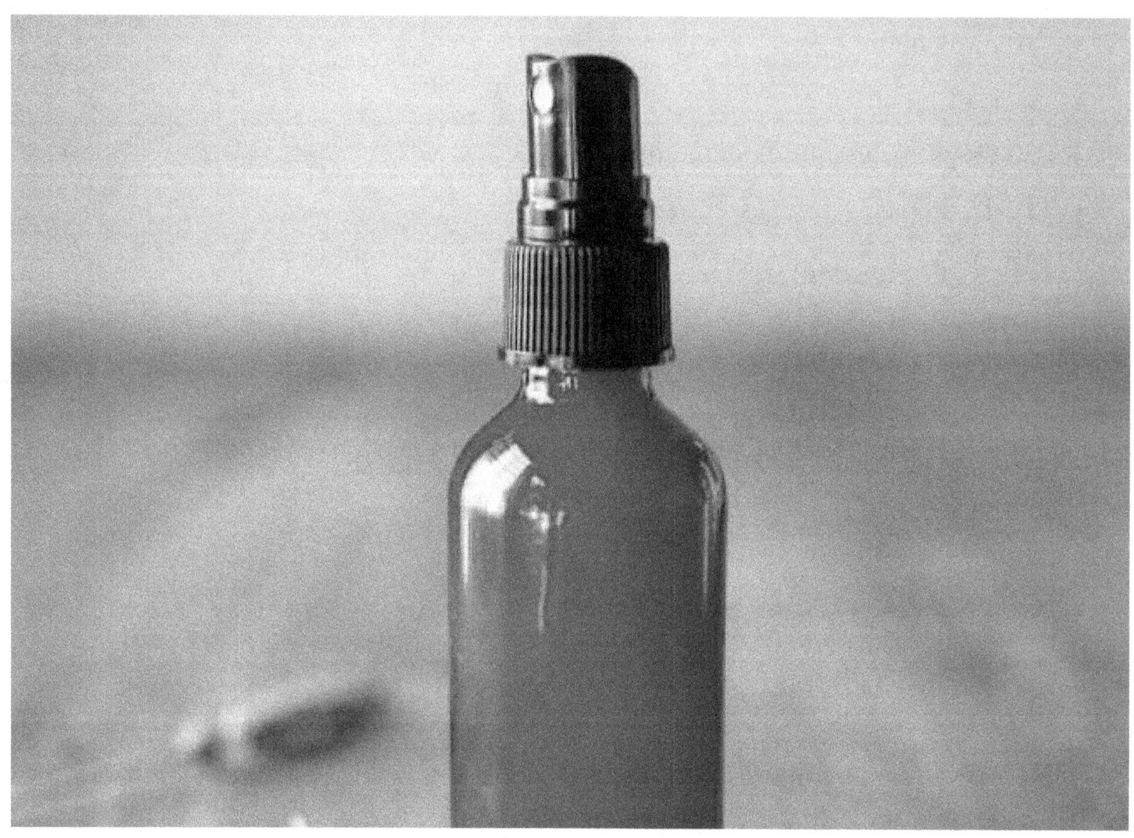

Great smell for small spaces; makes approx. 13-16 oz.

Ingredients:

- 3 oz sterile water
- 10 oz alcohol
- ¼-1/3 tsp peroxide
- 10-15 drops sage essential oil
- 15-20 drops lavender essential oil
- 5 drops green food coloring

Instructions:

In a spray bottle mix together water, alcohol, peroxide, sage & lavender oils, green food coloring.

Eucalyptus & Rose Disinfecting Spray for High Traffic Areas

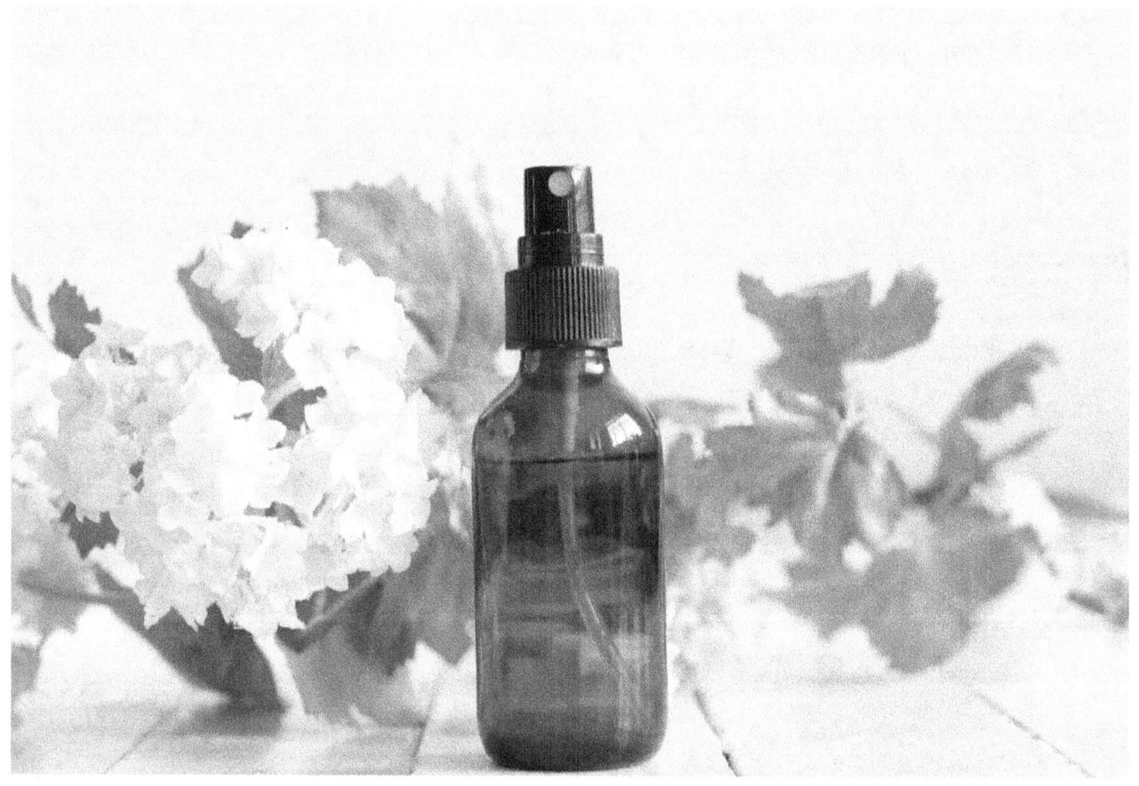

Great for living rooms and bedrooms; makes approx. 13-16 oz.

Ingredients:

- 3 oz sterile water
- 10 oz alcohol
- ¼-1/3 tsp peroxide
- 20 drops eucalyptus essential oil
- 10-12 drops rose essential oil
- 3-4 drops purple or red drops of food coloring

Instructions:

In a spray bottle mix together water, alcohol, peroxide, eucalyptus & rose oil, blue food coloring.

Lemon-Sage Disinfecting Spray

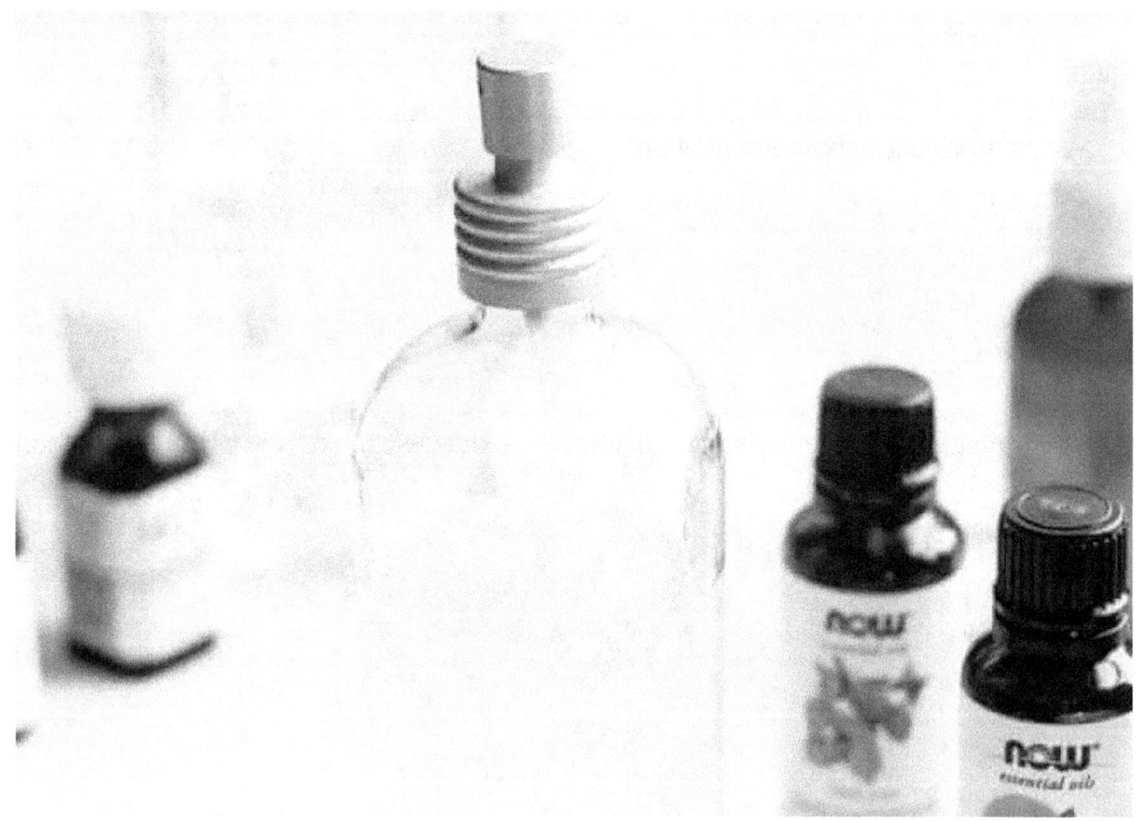

Safe around pets! makes approx. 13-16 oz.

Ingredients:

- 3 oz sterile water
- 10 oz alcohol
- ¼-1/3 tsp peroxide
- 20 drops lemon essential oil
- 10 drops sage essential oil
- 3-4 drops yellow food coloring

Instructions:

In a spray bottle mix together water, alcohol, peroxide, lemon & sage, yellow food coloring.

Lemon DIY Disinfecting Wipes with Isopropyl Alcohol

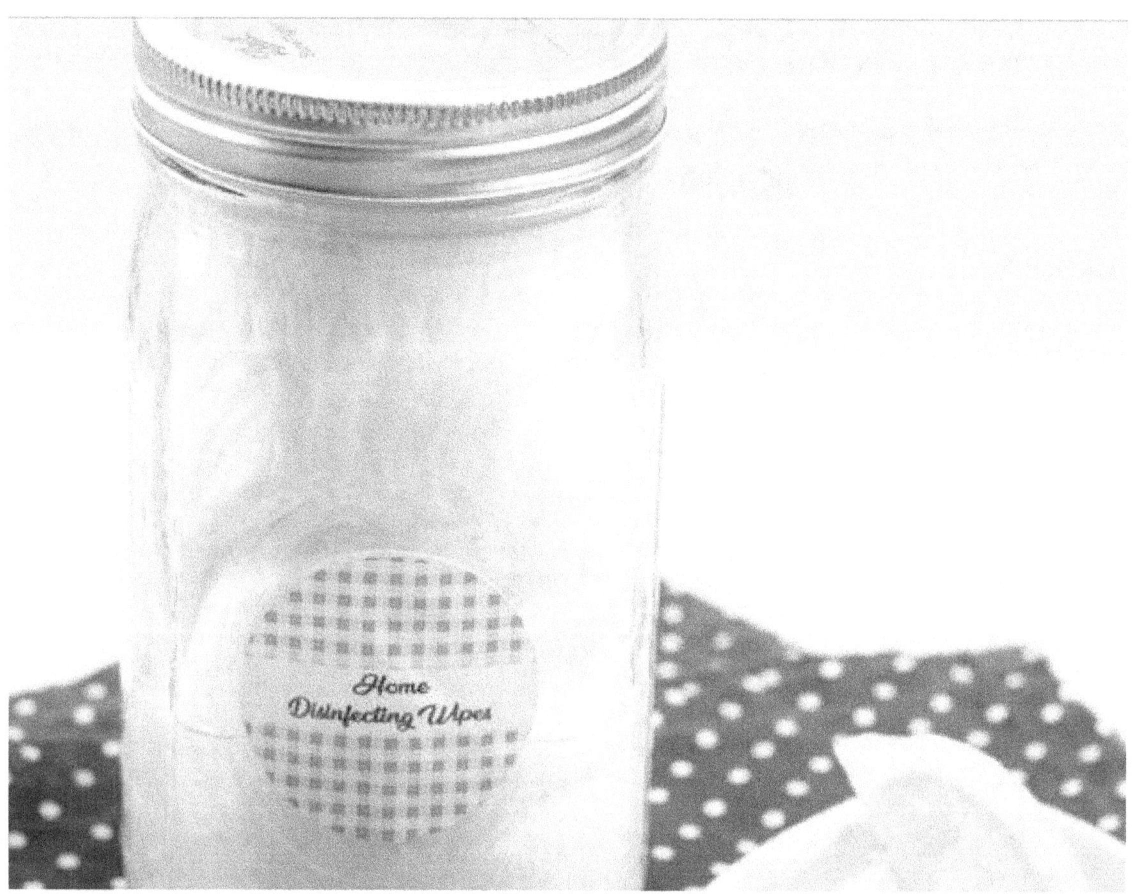

Great to keep in bedrooms! Makes approx. 150-180 wipes.

Ingredients:

- 16-18 oz 91-99% isopropyl alcohol
- 3-5 oz sterile water
- 1 ½ tsp peroxide
- 25-30 drops lemon essential oil

Instructions:

Mix together alcohol, water, peroxide, lemon essential oil. Submerge papers towels into mixture. Let drain and stick inside a jar or container.

Lemon DIY Disinfecting Wipes with Ethanol Alcohol

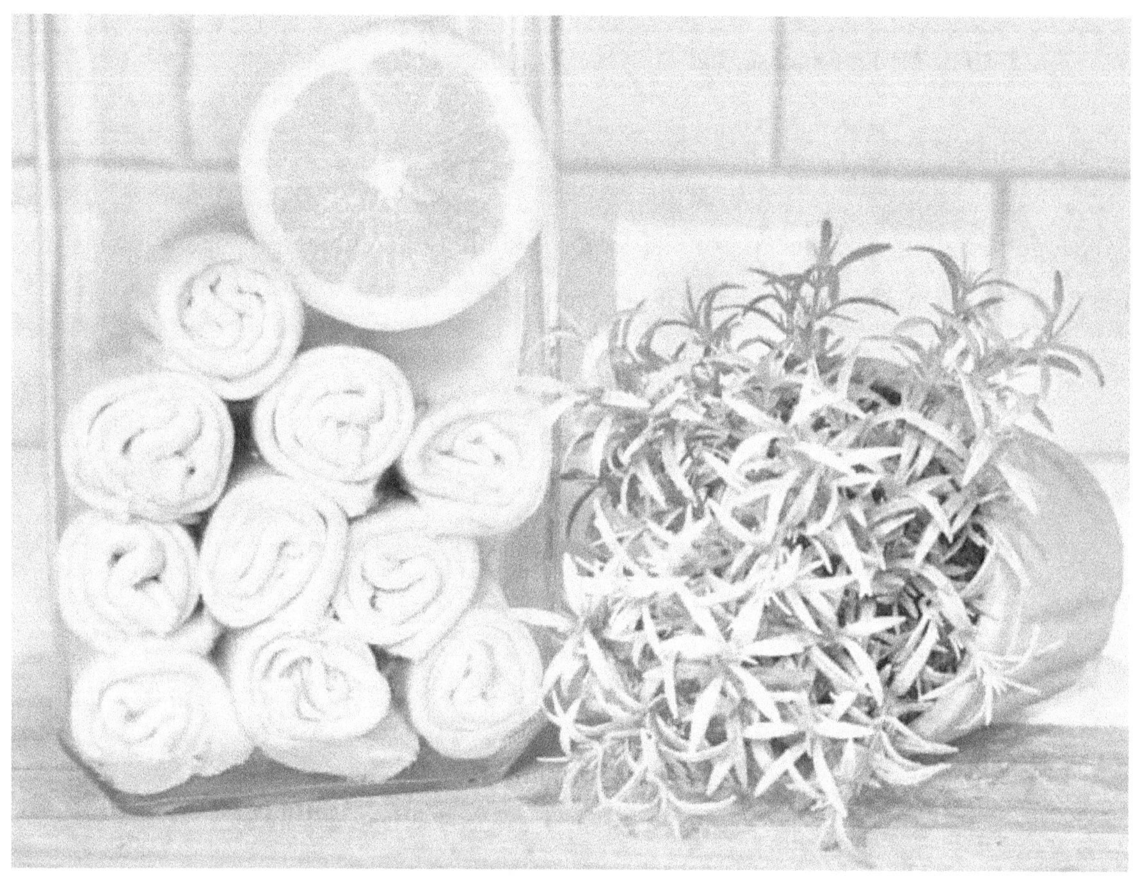

Don't forget remotes! Makes approx. 150-180 wipes.

Ingredients:

- 16-18 oz ethanol alcohol
- 1-2 oz sterile water
- 25-30 drops of lemon essential oil

Instructions:

Mix together alcohol, water, lemon essential oil. Submerge papers towels into mixture. Let drain and stick inside a jar or container.

Lemon Thyme Disinfecting Wipes with Isopropyl Alcohol

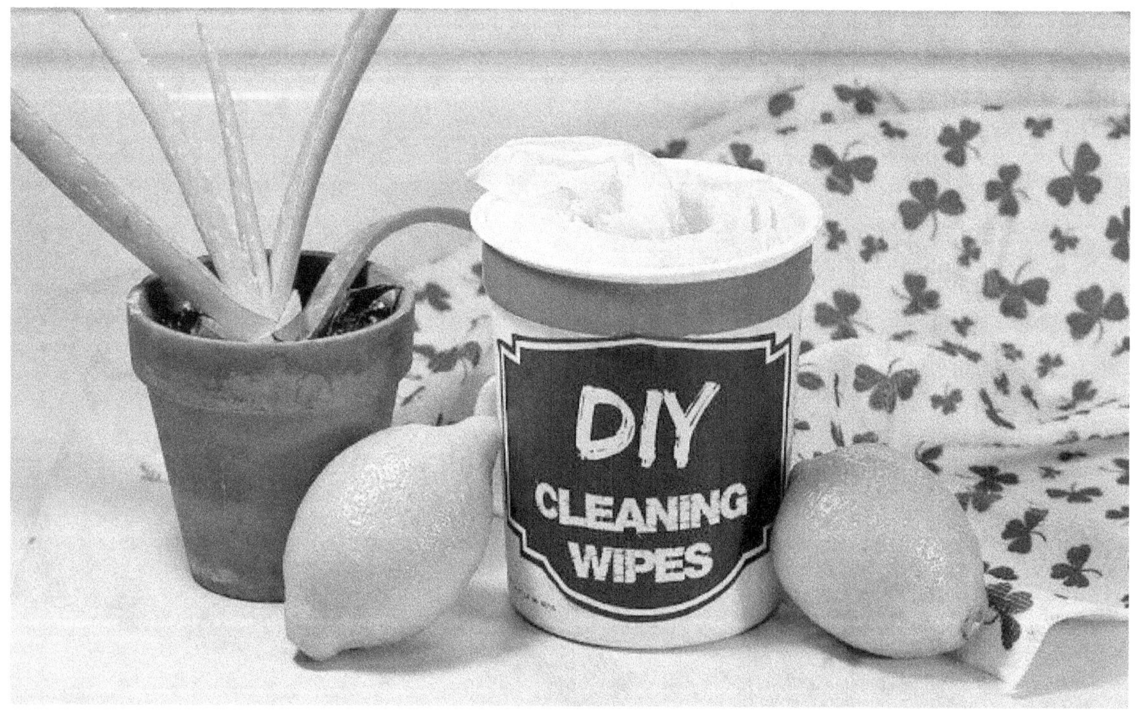

Great to keep in purses or backpacks! Makes approx. 150-180 wipes.

Ingredients:

- 16-18 oz 91-99% isopropyl alcohol
- 3-5 oz sterile water
- 1 ½ tsp peroxide
- 20 drops lemon essential oil
- 10-12 drops thyme essential oil

Instructions:

Mix together alcohol, water, peroxide, lemon & thyme essential oils. Submerge papers towels into mixture. Let drain and stick inside a jar or container.

Lemon-Thyme Disinfecting Car Wipes with Ethanol Alcohol

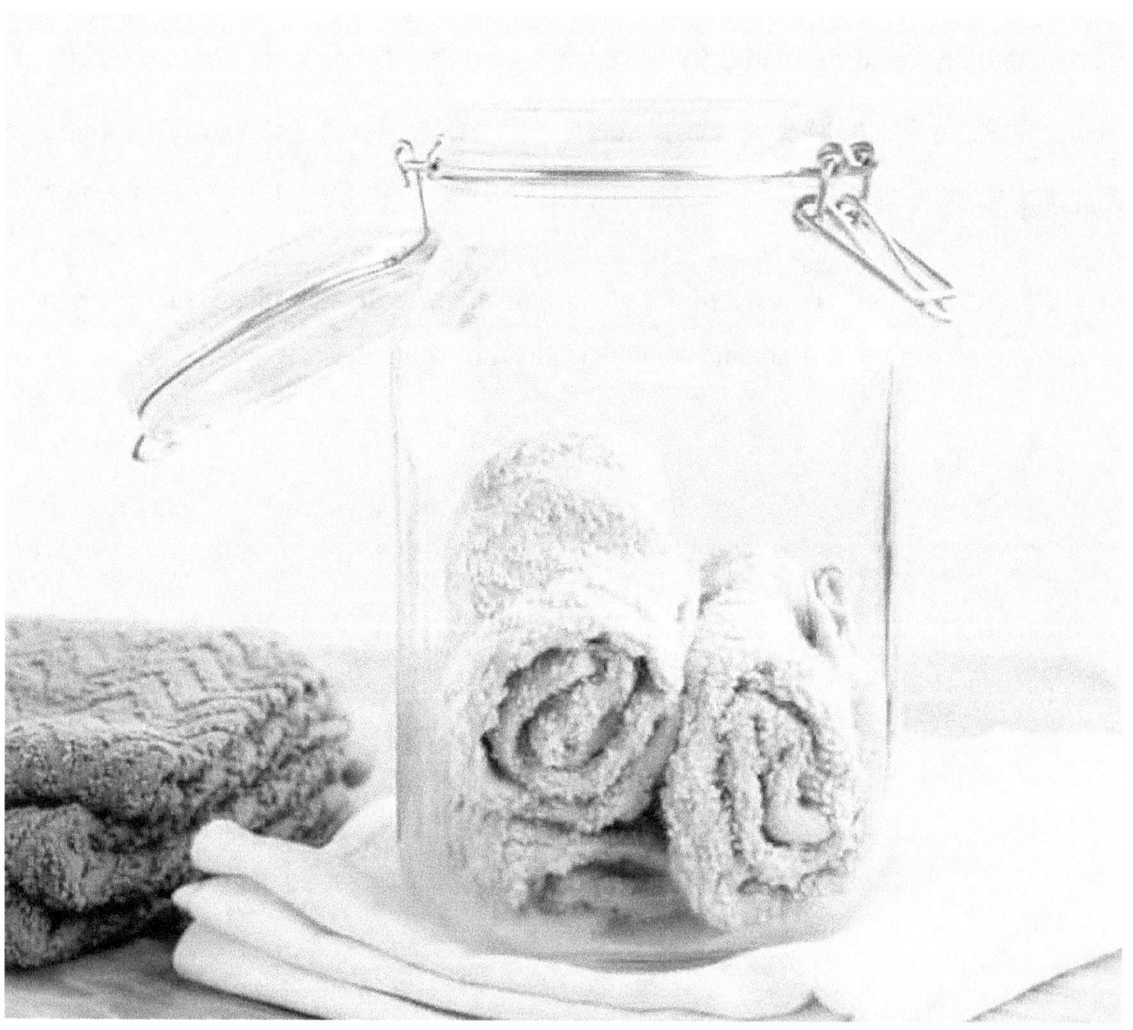

Good for cars! Makes approx. 150-180 wipes.

Ingredients:

- 16-18 oz ethanol alcohol
- 1-2 oz sterile water
- 20-25 drops lemon essential oil
- 10-15 drops thyme essential oil

Instructions:

Mix together alcohol, water, lemon & thyme essential oils. Submerge papers towels into mixture. Let drain and stick inside a jar or container.

Lemon Rose Power Wipes with Isopropyl Alcohol

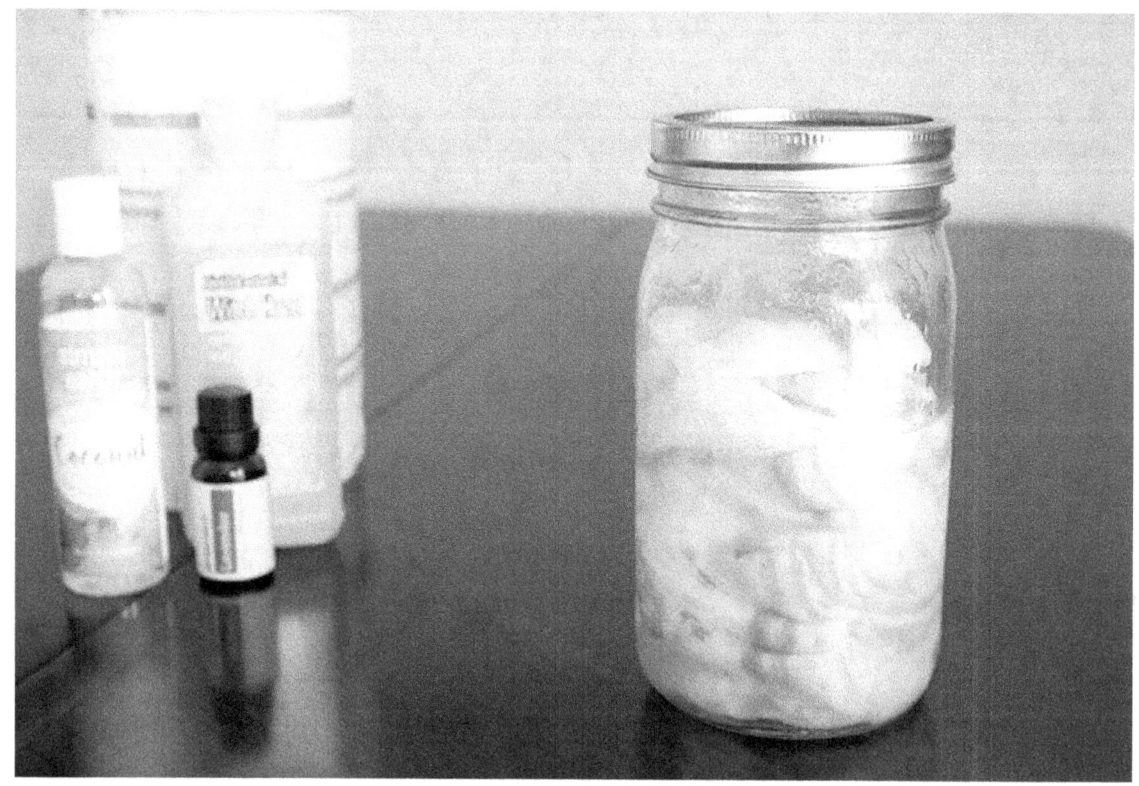

Great multi-purpose wipe! Makes approx. 150-180 wipes.

Ingredients:

- 16-18 oz 91-99% isopropyl alcohol
- 3-5 oz sterile water
- 1 ½ tsp peroxide
- 20 drops lemon essential oil
- 10 drops rose essential oil
- 2-3 drops red or purple food coloring

Instructions:

Mix together alcohol, water, peroxide, lemon & rose essential oil, food coloring. Submerge paper towels into mixture. Let drain and stick inside a jar or container.

DIY Multi-Purpose Disinfecting Wipes with Ethanol Alcohol

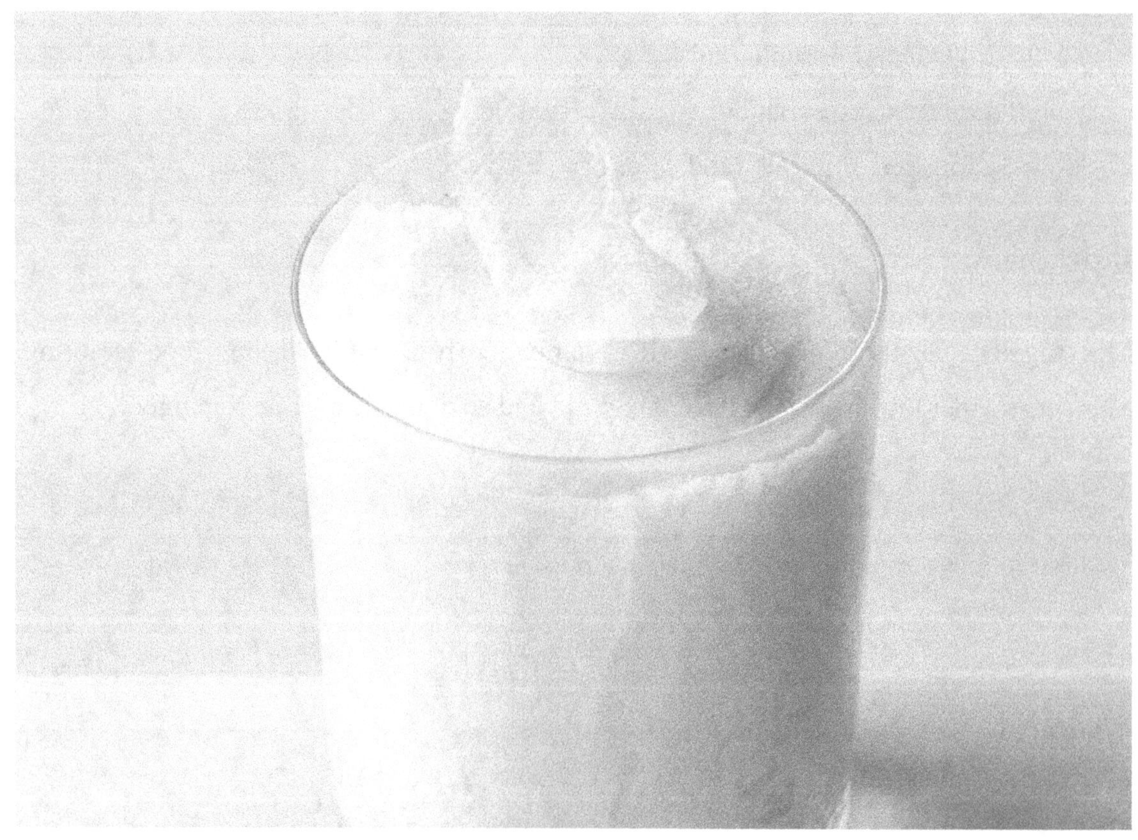

Clean everything! Makes approx. 150-180 wipes.

Ingredients:

- 16-18 oz ethanol alcohol
- 1-2 oz sterile water
- 20 drops rose essential oil
- 5-7 drops tea tree oil

Instructions:

Mix together alcohol, water, rose & tea tree essential oils. Submerge papers towels into mixture. Let drain and stick inside a jar or container.

DIY Easy Extra Strength Disinfecting Wipes

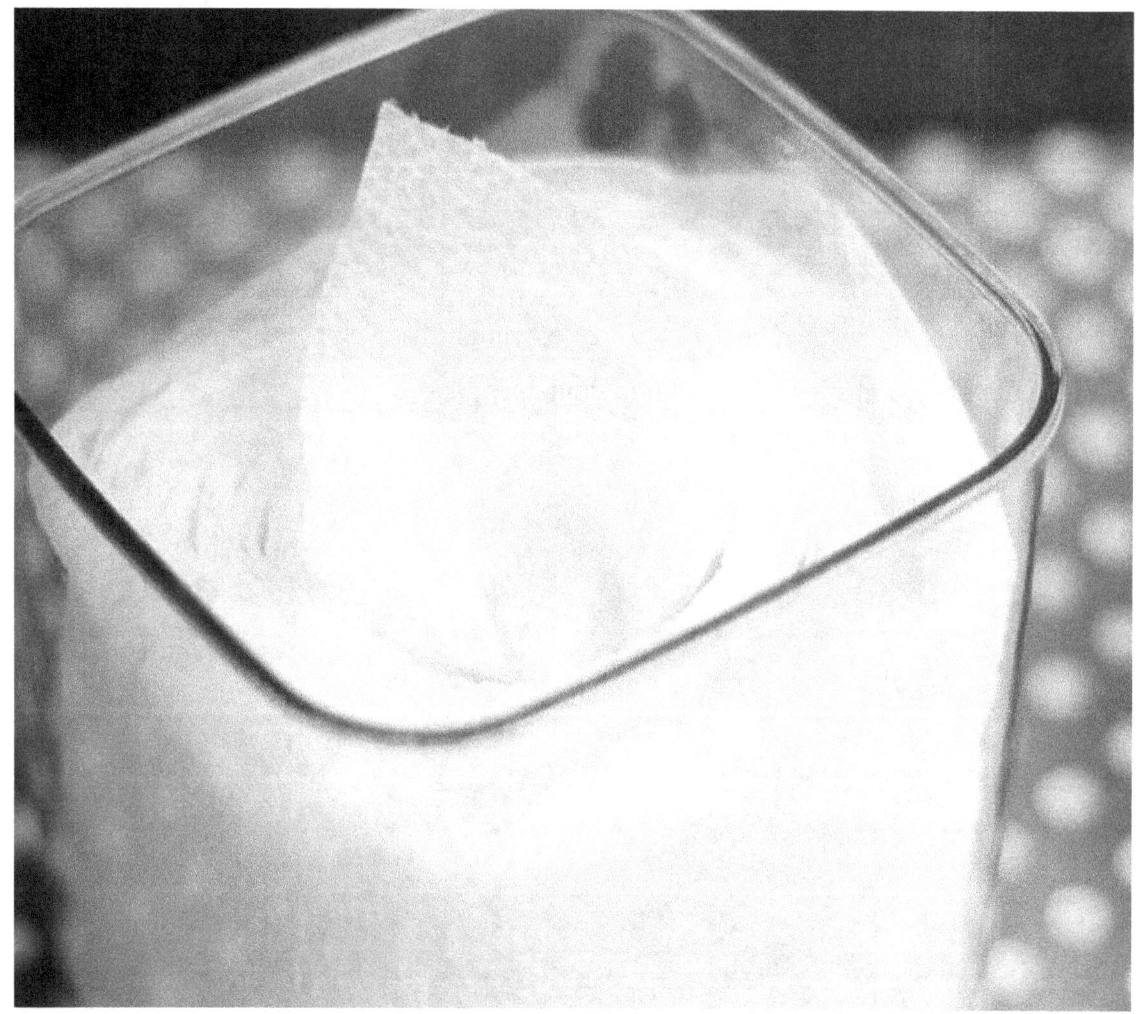

Great for the gym! Makes approx. 150-180 wipes.

Ingredients:

- 16-18 oz 91-99% isopropyl alcohol
- 3-5 oz sterile water
- 1 ½ tsp peroxide
- 5-10 drops tea tree oil

Instructions:

Mix together alcohol, water, peroxide, tea tree oil. Submerge paper towels into mixture. Let drain and stick inside a jar or container.

Extra Strength Disinfecting Wipes with Ethanol Alcohol

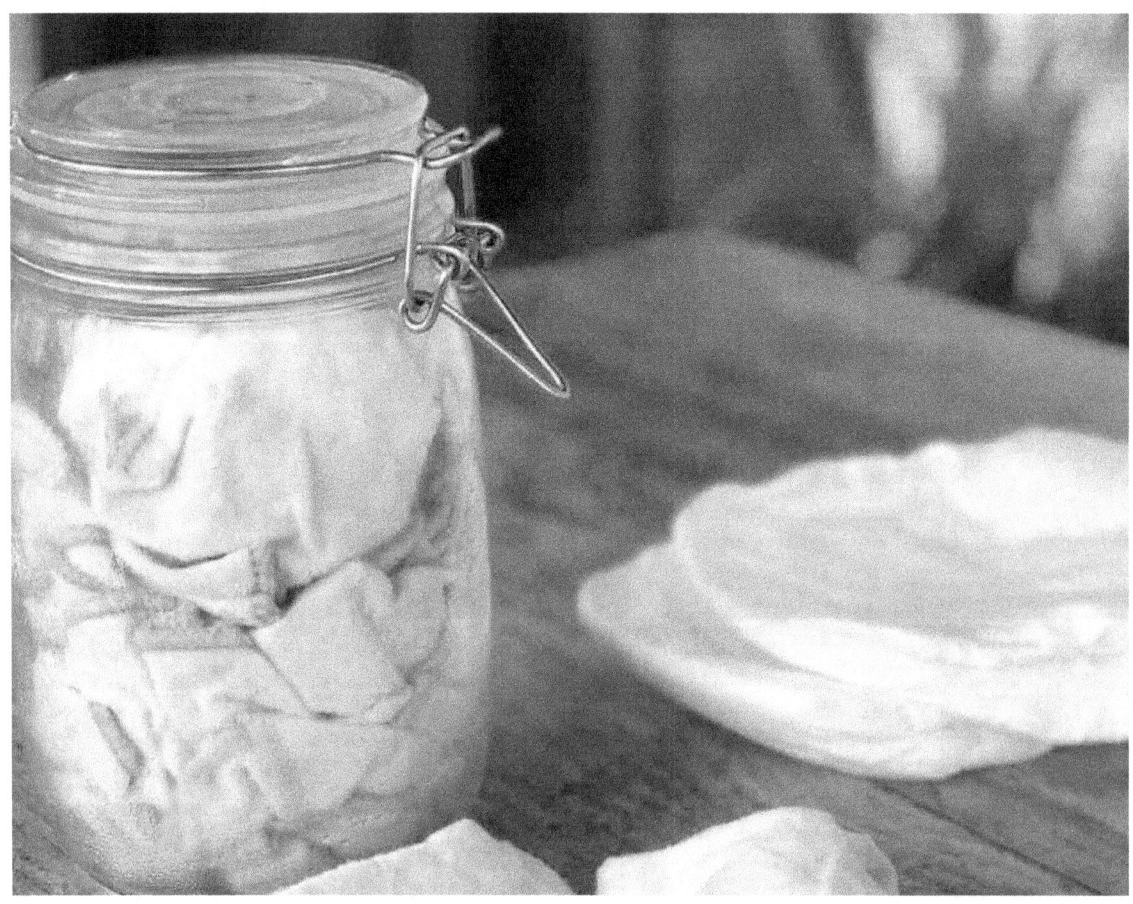

Great for extra germy surfaces! Makes approx. 150-180 wipes.

Ingredients:

- 16-18 oz ethanol alcohol
- 1-2 oz sterile water
- 5-7 drops tea tree oil

Instructions:

Mix together alcohol, water, tea tree oil. Submerge paper towels into mixture. Let drain and stick inside a jar or container.

Easy DIY All-Purpose Cleaner with Vodka

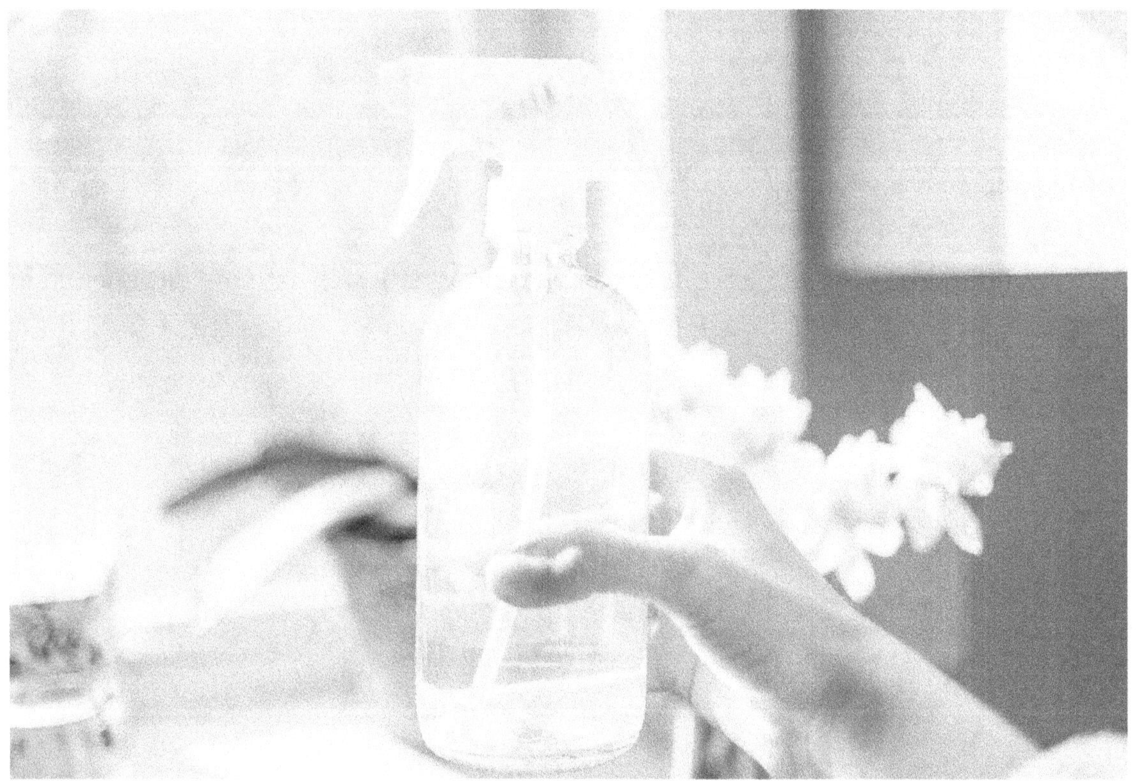

Easy! Makes 1 spray bottle.

Ingredients:

- 1/3 of bottle with vodka
- ¼-1/3 of bottle with sterile hot water
- ¼-1/3 of bottle with distilled vinegar
- 20-40 drops of thyme or tea tree oil

Instructions:

Mix all ingredients in spray bottle and shake.

Easy DIY All-Purpose Cleaner Wipes with Vodka

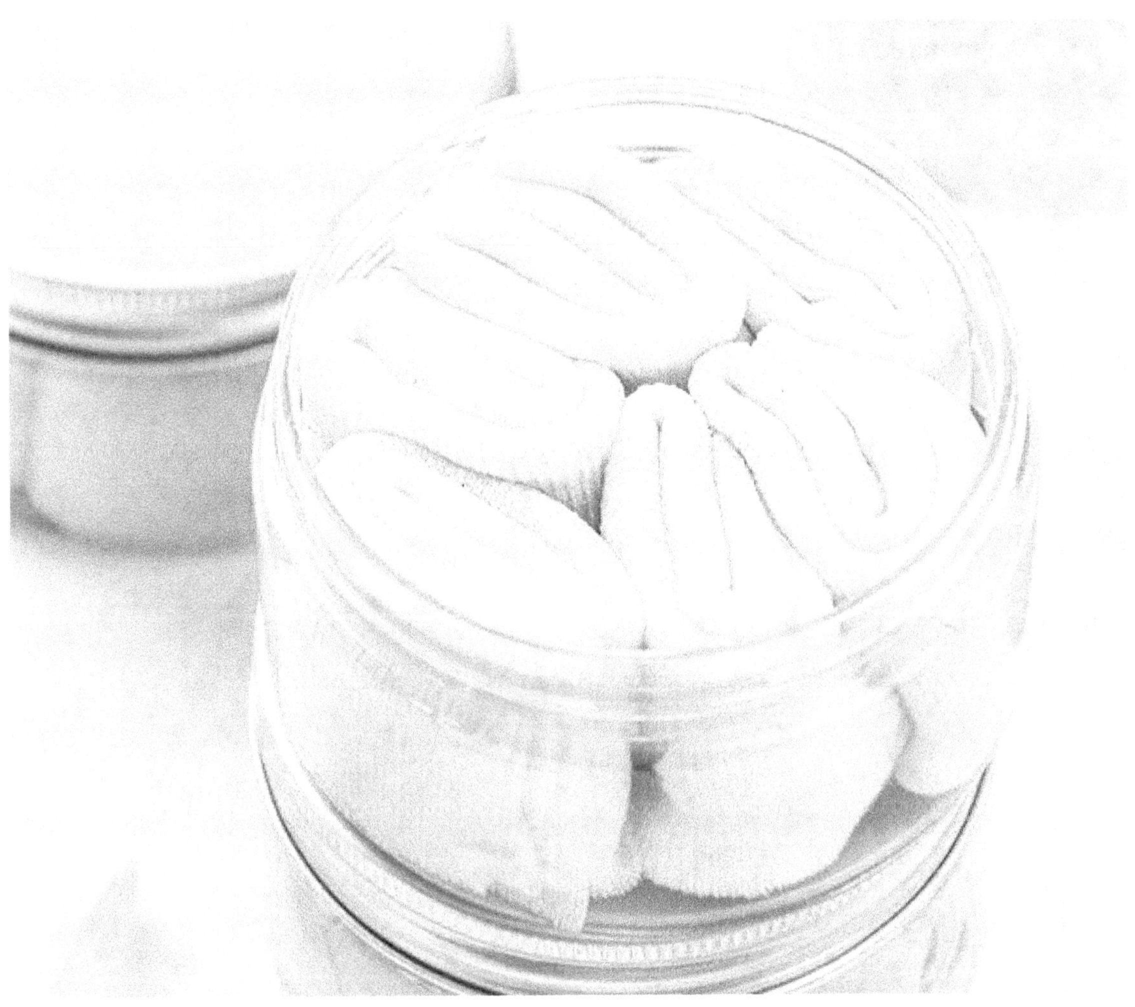

Easy to remember formula! Makes 150-180 wipes.

Ingredients:

- 2/3 cup vodka
- ¼ cup sterile hot water
- 1/3 of bottle with distilled vinegar
- 20-40 drops of thyme or tea tree oil

Instructions:

Mix all ingredients together in bowl.

Submerge paper towels in mixture.

Place wipes in a container.

Will keep 2-4 weeks.

DIY Kitchen All-Purpose Cleaner Wipes with Vodka

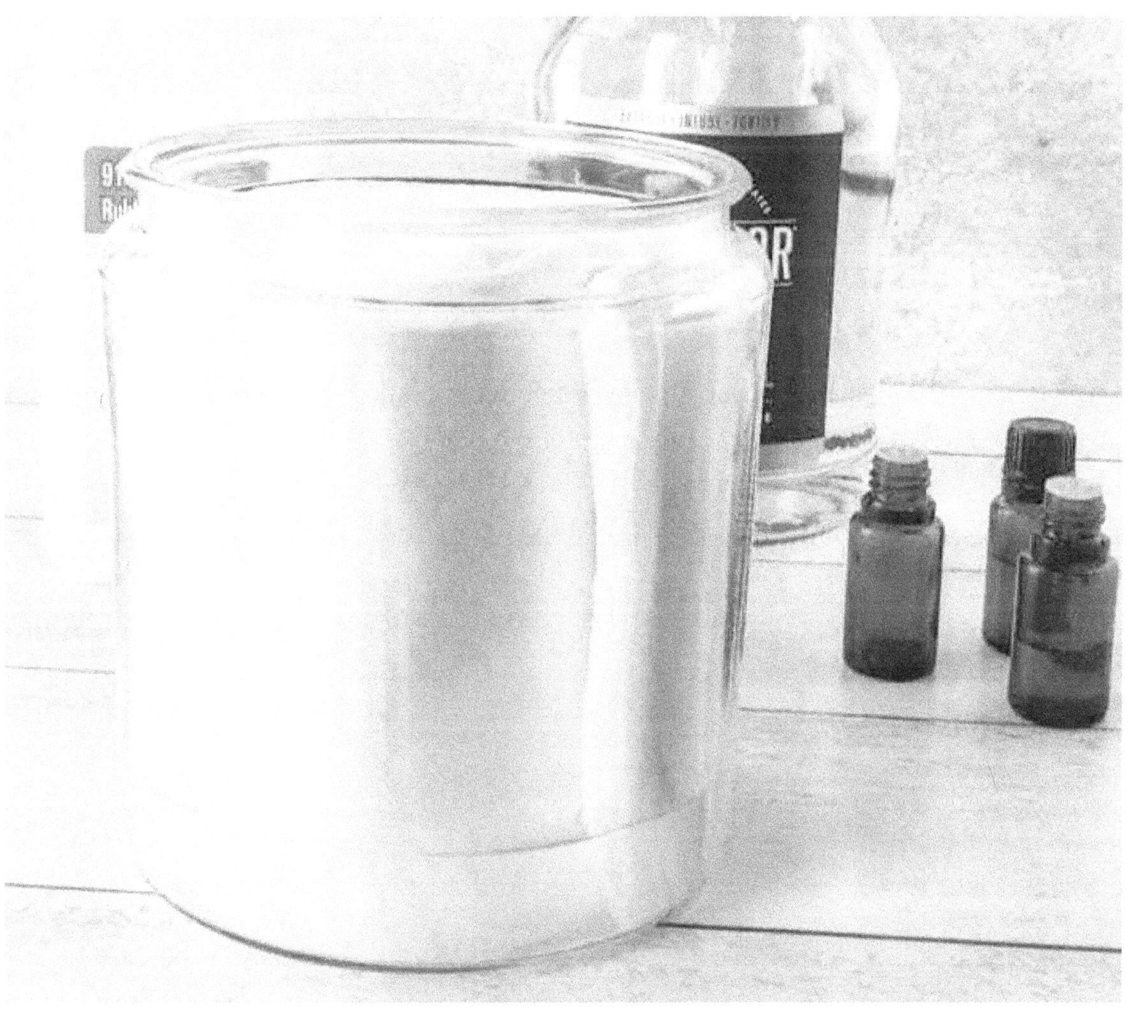

Great for bathrooms too! Makes 150-180 wipes.

Ingredients:

- 2/3 cup vodka
- ¼ cup sterile hot water
- 1/3 of bottle with distilled vinegar
- 15 drops of thyme or tea tree oil
- 20-30 lemon essential oil

Instructions:

Mix vodka, sterile water, vinegar, thyme or tea tree oil, and lemon essential oil together in bowl.

Submerge paper towels in mixture.

Place wipes in a container.

Will keep 2-4 weeks.

DIY Disinfectant Spray for Granite Counters

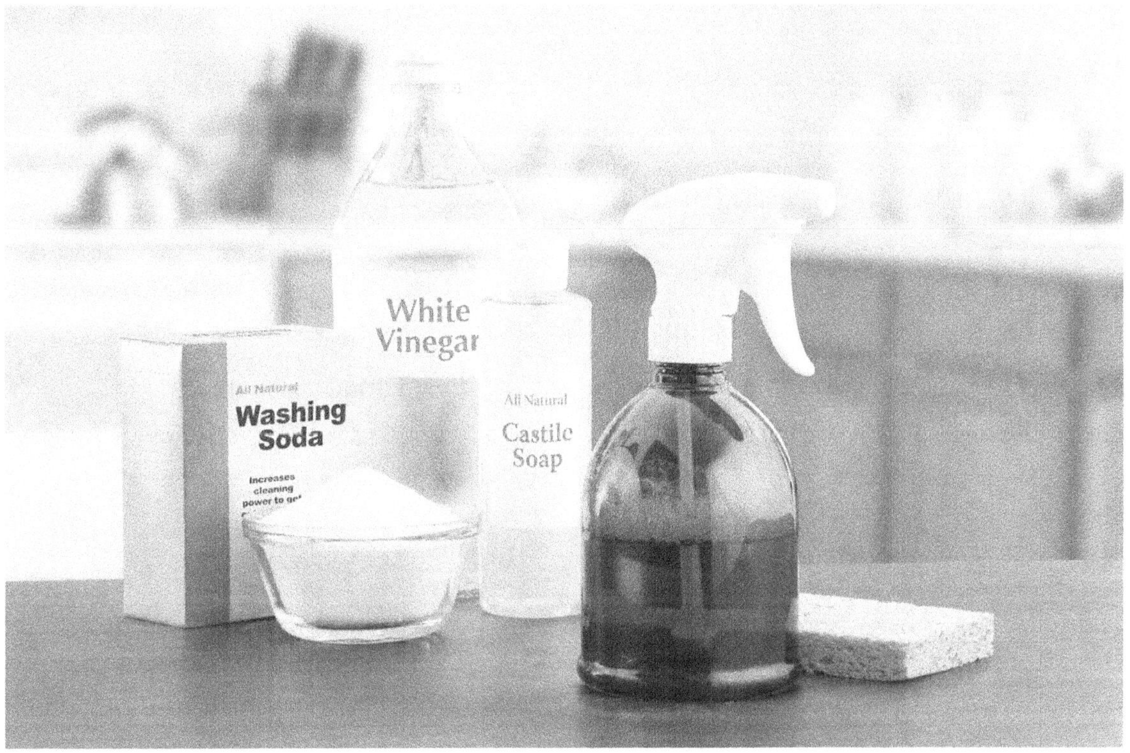

Granite tough but safe! Makes 8-24 oz.

Ingredients:

- ¼ cup 70% isopropyl alcohol
- 1/3 tsp dish soap (example: Dawn)
- 14-1/3 cup sterile water
- 5-10 drops thyme or tea tree oil
- 15-20 drops lemon essential oil

Instructions:

In bottle mix together alcohol, dish soap, water, thyme & lemon essential oils.

DIY Disinfectant Wipes for Granite Counters

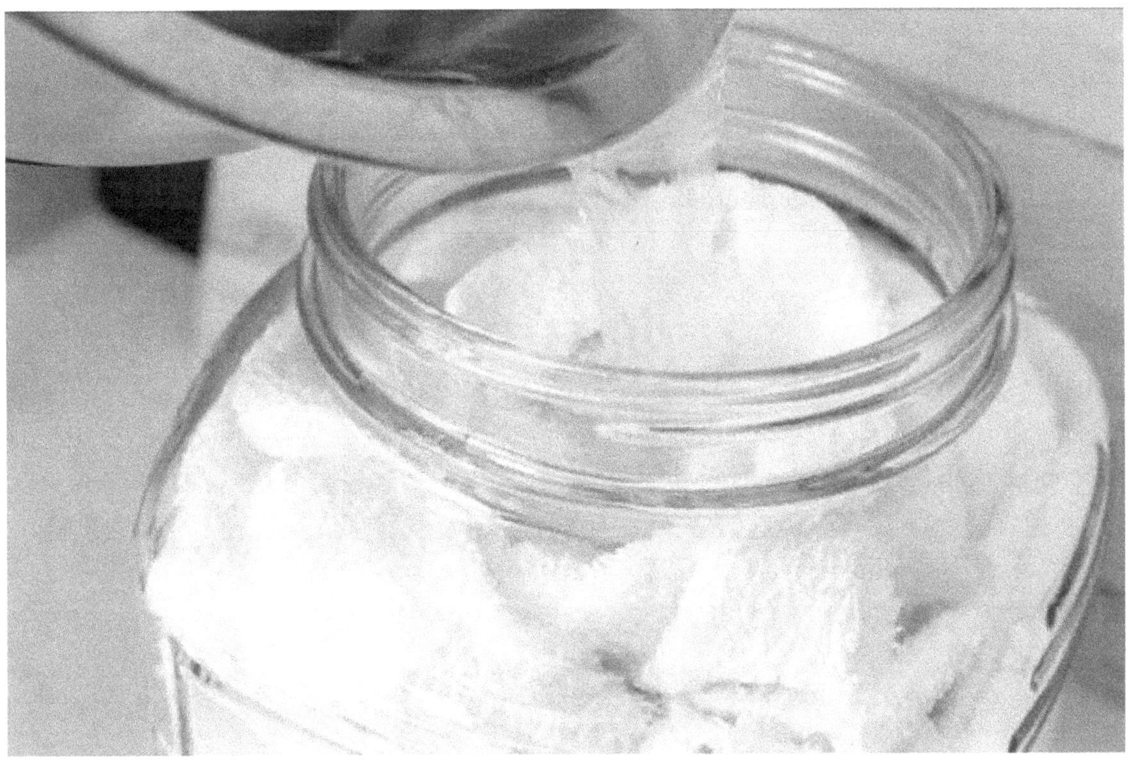

For quick clean ups! Makes 150-180 wipes

Ingredients:

- ¼ cup 70% isopropyl alcohol
- 1/3 tsp dish soap (example: Dawn)
- 14-1/3 cup sterile water
- 5-10 drops thyme or tea tree oil
- 15-20 drops lemon essential oil

Instructions:

In bottle mix together alcohol, dish soap, water, thyme & lemon essential oils.

Submerge both halves of towels in mixture.

Place wipes in a container

L & L Disinfectant Wipes for Granite Counters

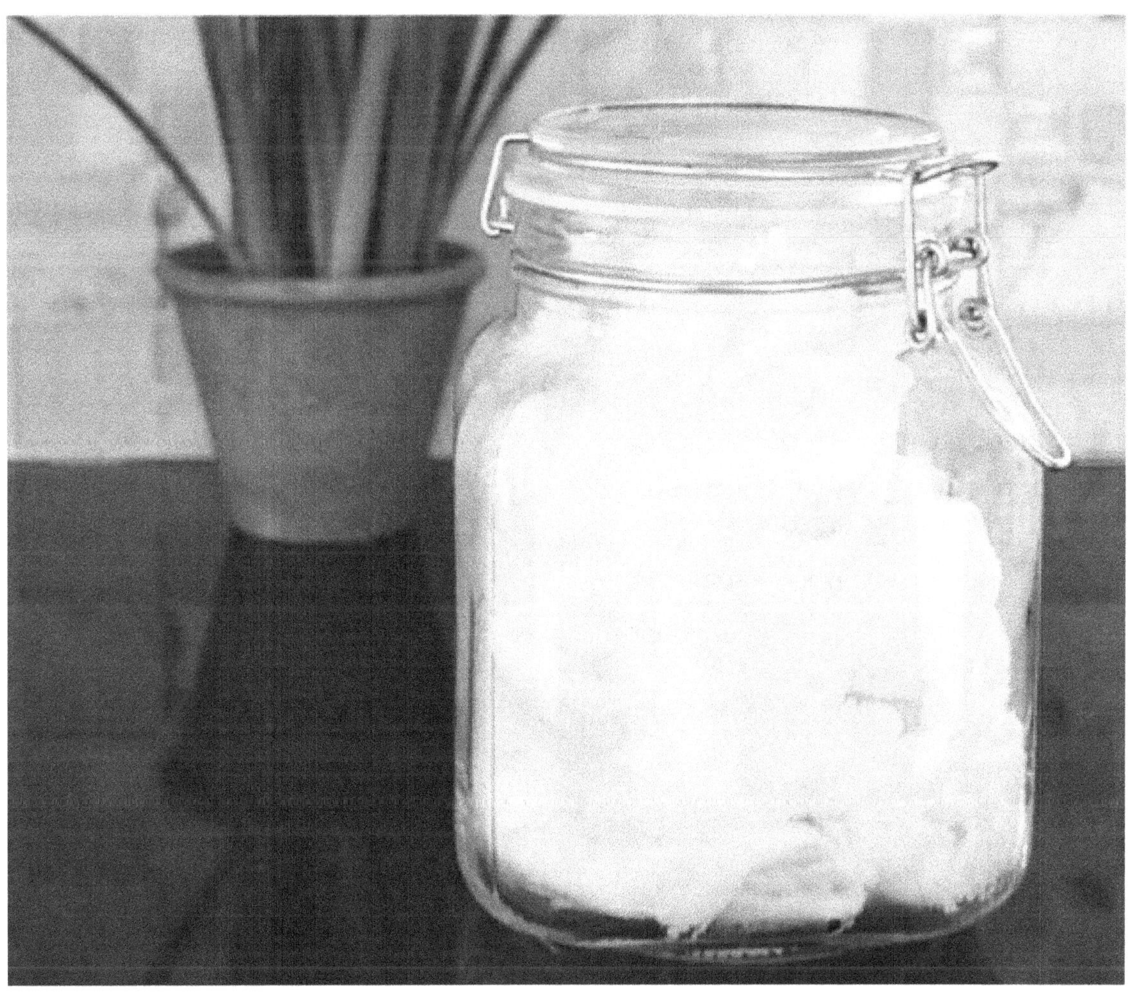

A relaxing scent! Makes 150-180 wipes

Ingredients:

- ¼ cup 70% isopropyl alcohol
- 1/3 tsp dish soap (example: Dawn)
- 14-1/3 cup sterile water
- 5-10 drops lavender essential oil
- 15-20 drops lemon essential oil

Instructions:

In bottle mix together alcohol, dish soap, water, lavender & lemon essential oils.

Submerge both halves of towels in mixture.

Place wipes in a container

Grapefruit Disinfectant Wipes for Granite Counters

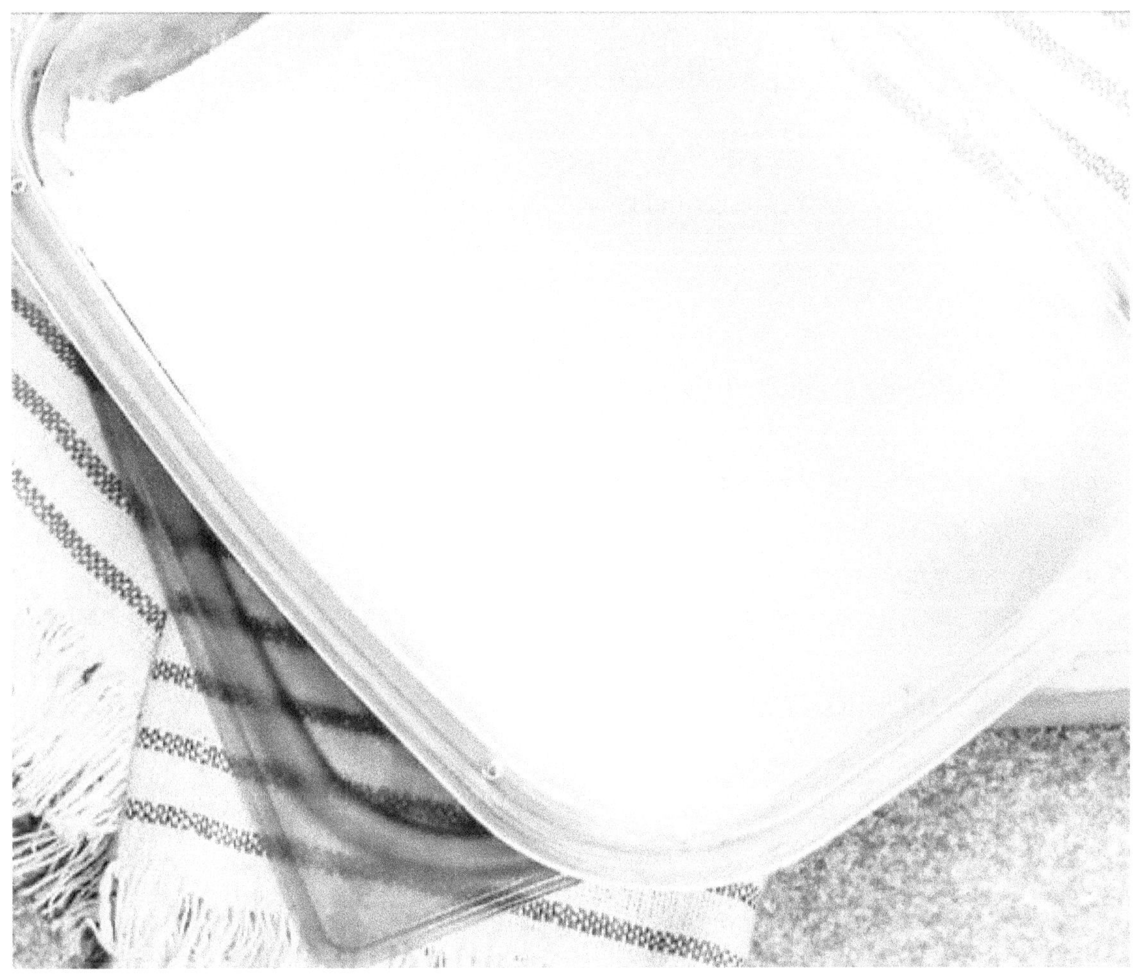

Great for bathroom ! Makes 150-180 wipes

Ingredients:

- ¼ cup 70% isopropyl alcohol
- 1/3 tsp dish soap (example: Dawn)
- 14-1/3 cup sterile water
- 5-10 drops thyme or tea tree oil
- 15-20 drops grapefruit essential oil

Instructions:

In bottle mix together alcohol, dish soap, water, thyme & grapefruit essential oils.

Submerge both halves of towels in mixture.

Place wipes in a container.

Orange-Sage Disinfectant Spray for Granite Counters

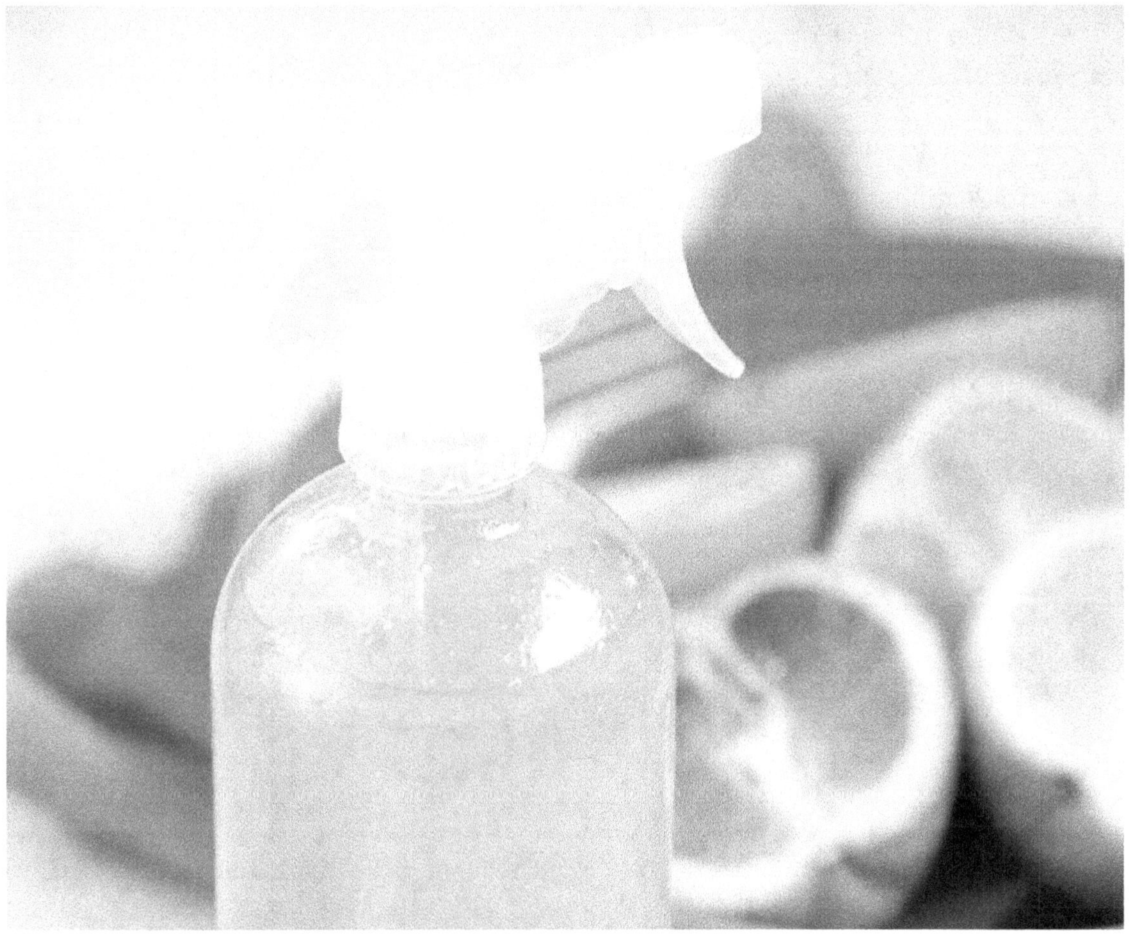

For quick clean ups! Makes 8-16 oz

Ingredients:

- ¼ cup 70% isopropyl alcohol
- 1/3 tsp dish soap (example: Dawn)
- 14-1/3 cup sterile water
- 5-10 drops sage essential oil
- 15-20 drops orange essential oil

Instructions:

In bottle mix together alcohol, dish soap, water, orange & sage essential oils.

Easy Bleach Disinfectant

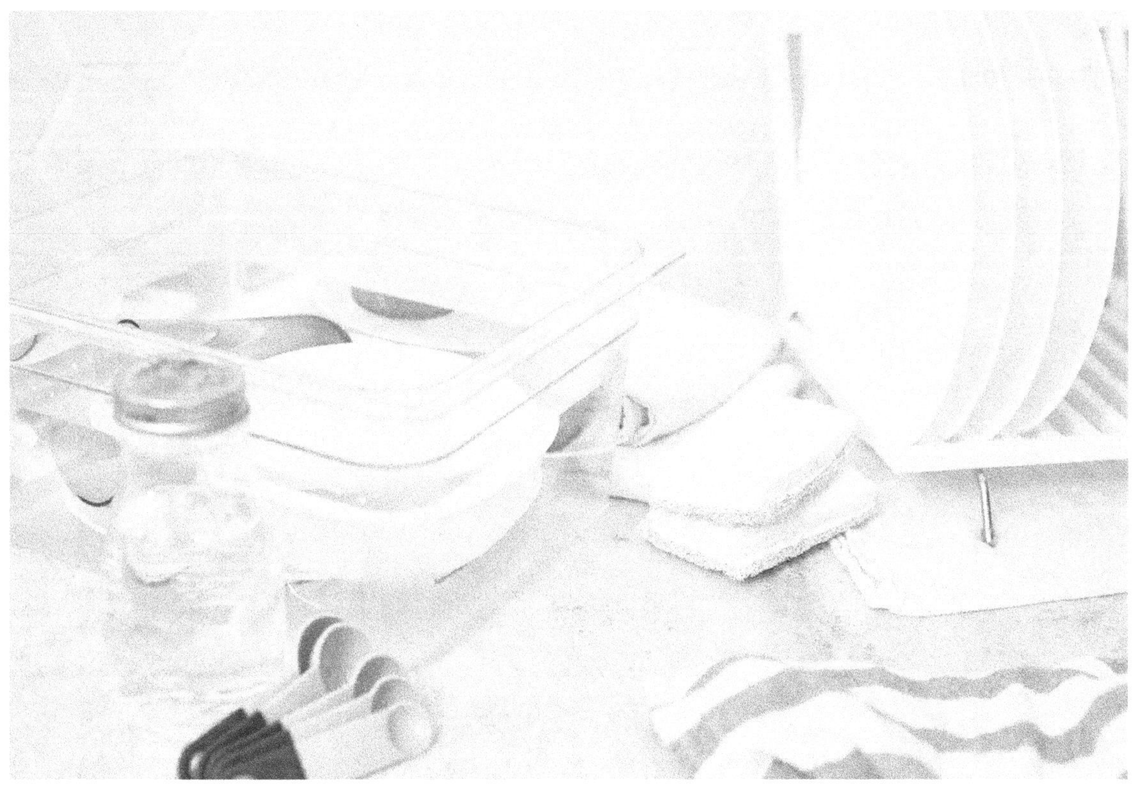

Kills virus! Recommended by the CDC! Makes 8-24 oz.

Ingredients:

- 1/3 cup bleach per gallon OR 4 teaspoons per quart

Instructions:

CDC states expired bleach will kill the virus.

Will stay good 1-2 days.

Let sit on surface 10 minutes.

Clorox Recommended Disinfect Spray

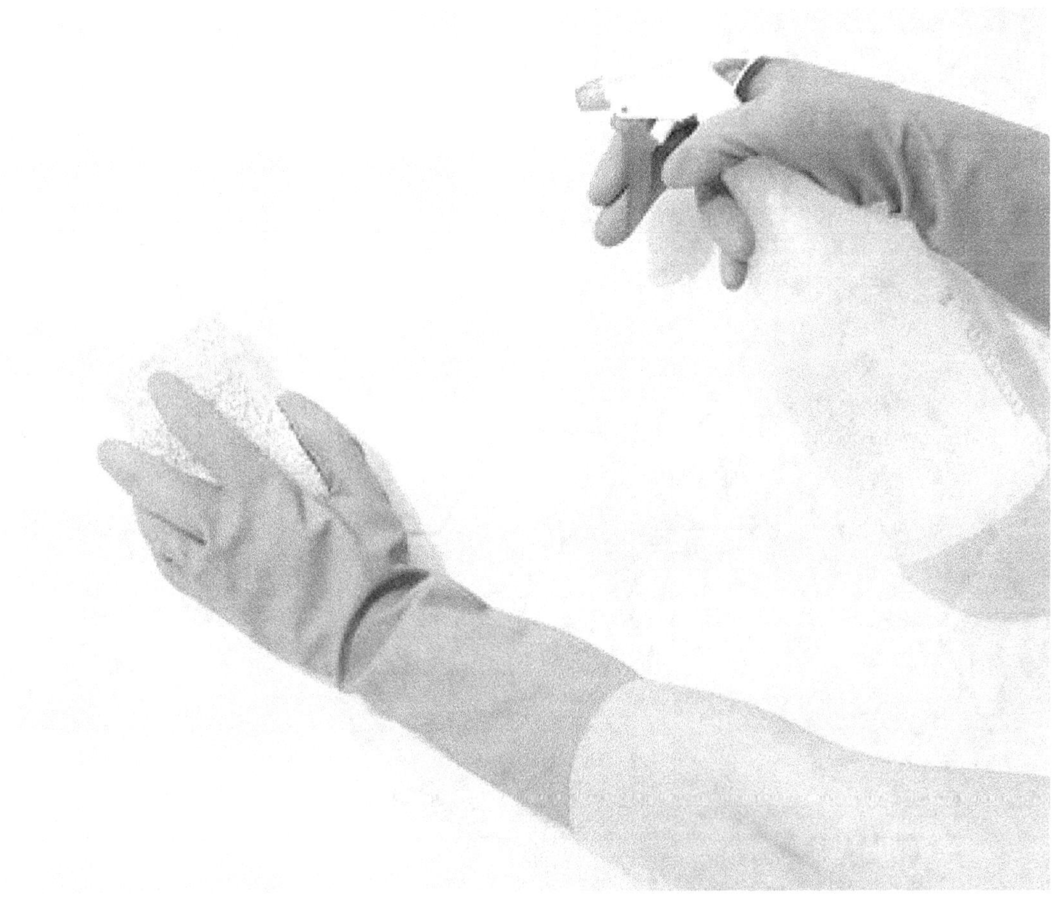

A little stronger than CDC recommendation! Makes 8-24 oz

Ingredients:

- ½ cup per gallon OR 2 Tbsp per quart

Instructions:

Let sit on surface 10 minutes.

DIY Bleach Wipes

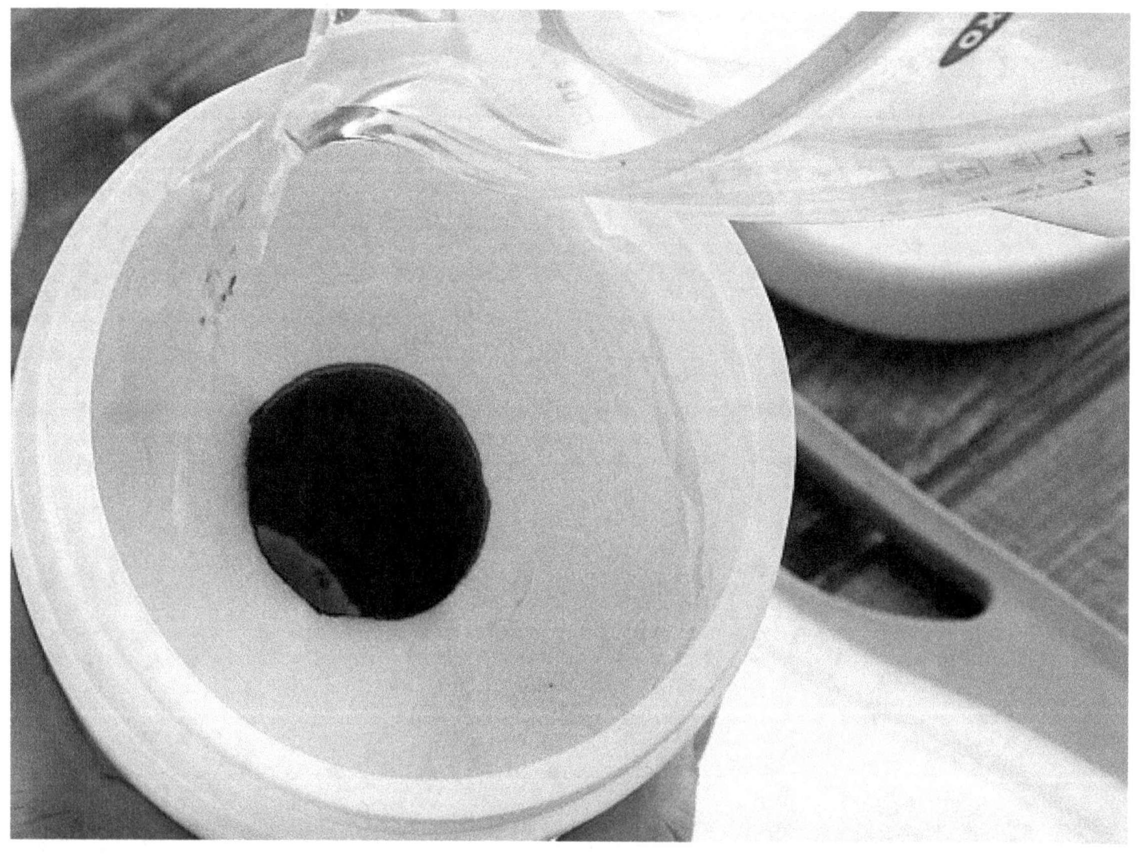

Be careful when working with bleach! Makes 150-180 wipes

Ingredients:

- 2 Tbsp bleach
- 2 1/3 cups water

Instructions:

In bowl mix together water and bleach.

Submerge paper towels into mixture.

Place towels into container.

Disinfecting Glass Cleaner

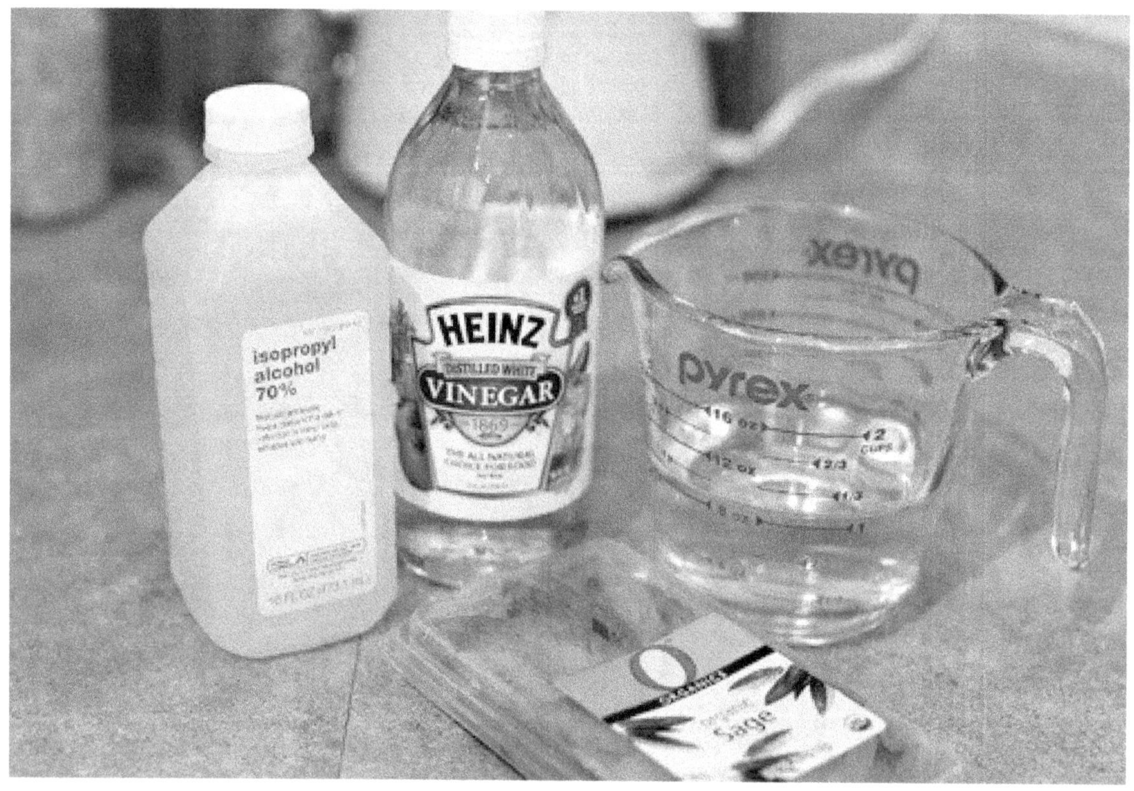

Great for cell phones! Makes 150-180 wipes

Ingredients:

- 1 ½ cup sterile water
- 2/3 cups rubbing alcohol
- ½ cup vinegar
- 2-4 drops blue food coloring

Instructions:

Mix together sterile water, rubbing alcohol, vinegar, food coloring in spray bottle.

Keep stored in a cool, dark place.

Homemade Anti-Bacterial Wipes

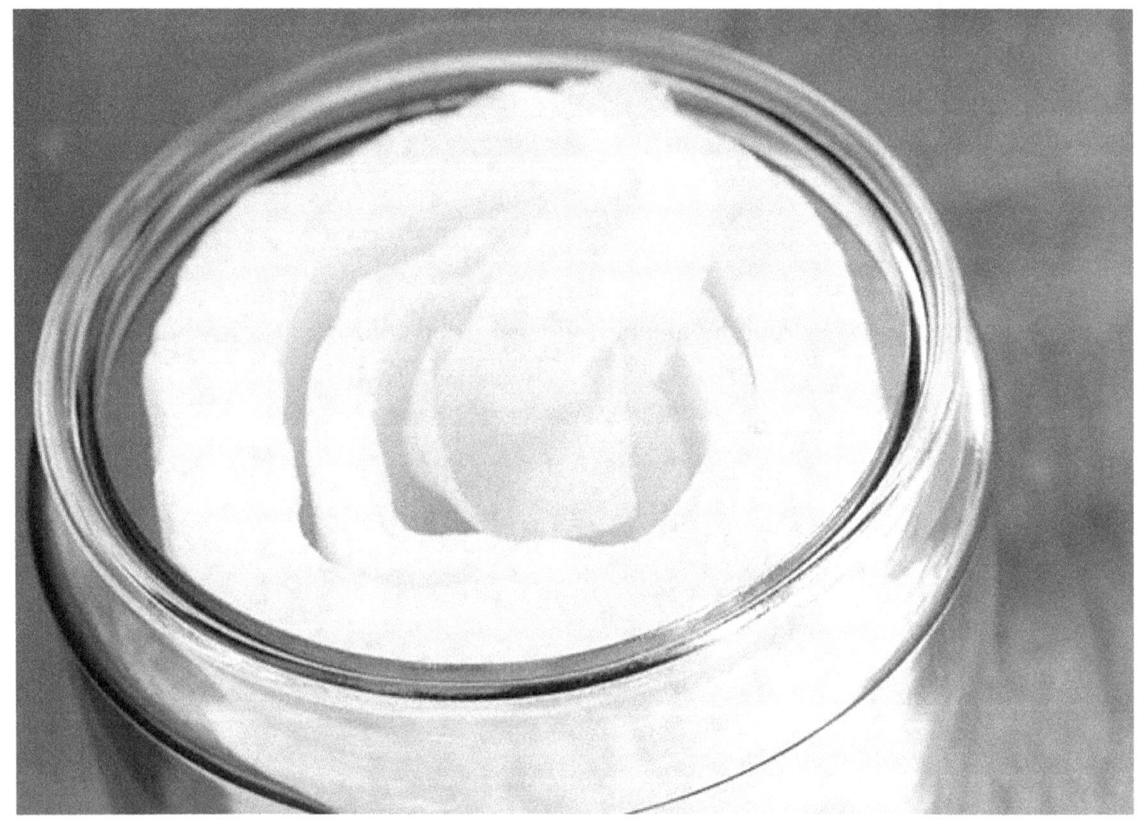

Use baby wipes! Makes 50 baby wipes or two small halves of a paper towel roll

Ingredients:

- 1 ½ cup 70% isopropyl alcohol or 140 proof vodka
- 1 Tbsp coconut oil
- 5-10 drops lavender essential oil
- 5-10 drops lemon essential oil

Instructions:

Mix together alcohol or vodka with coconut oil, lavender & lemon essential oil.

Submerge towel or wipes in mixture.

Place in a container.

Lemon & Coconut Disinfecting Wipes

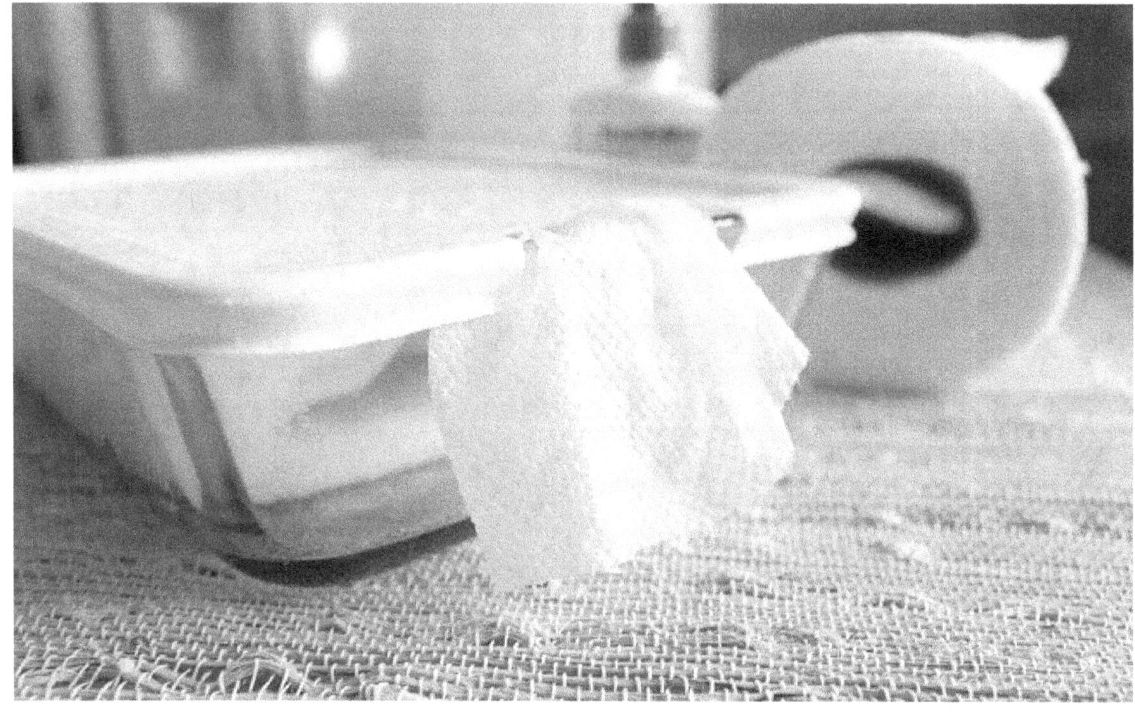

Great for kitchen spills! Makes 150-180 wipes

Ingredients:

- 1 ½ cup 70% isopropyl alcohol or 140 proof vodka
- 1 Tbsp coconut oil
- 20-30 drops lemon essential oil

Instructions:

Mix together alcohol or vodka with coconut oil, lavender & lemon essential oil.

Submerge towel or wipes in mixture.

Place in a container.

Lavender and Eucalyptus Disinfecting Wipes

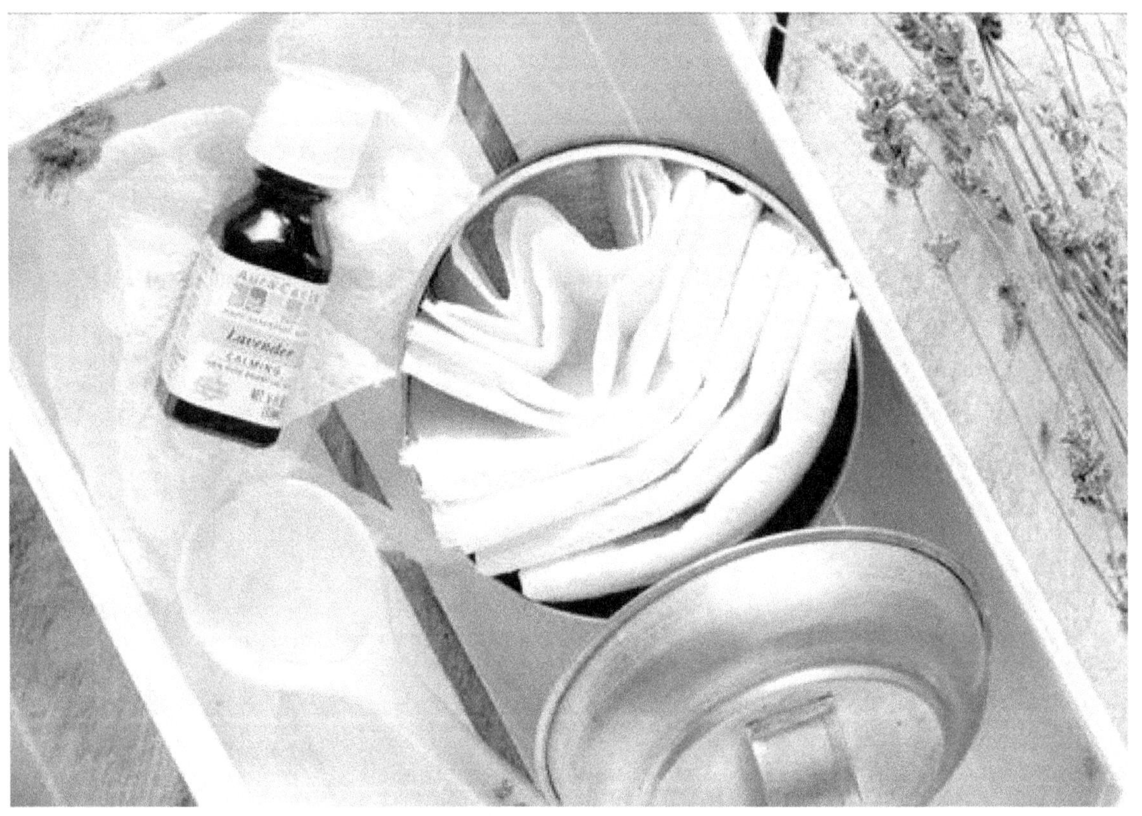

Use baby wipes! Makes 50 baby wipes or two small halves of a paper towel roll

Ingredients:

- 1 ½ cup 70% isopropyl alcohol or 140 proof vodka
- 1 Tbsp coconut oil
- 5-10 drops lavender essential oil
- 5-10 drops eucalyptus essential oil

Instructions:

Mix together alcohol or vodka with coconut oil, lavender & lemon essential oil.

Submerge towel or wipes in mixture.

Place in a container.

Cinna-mon Wipes

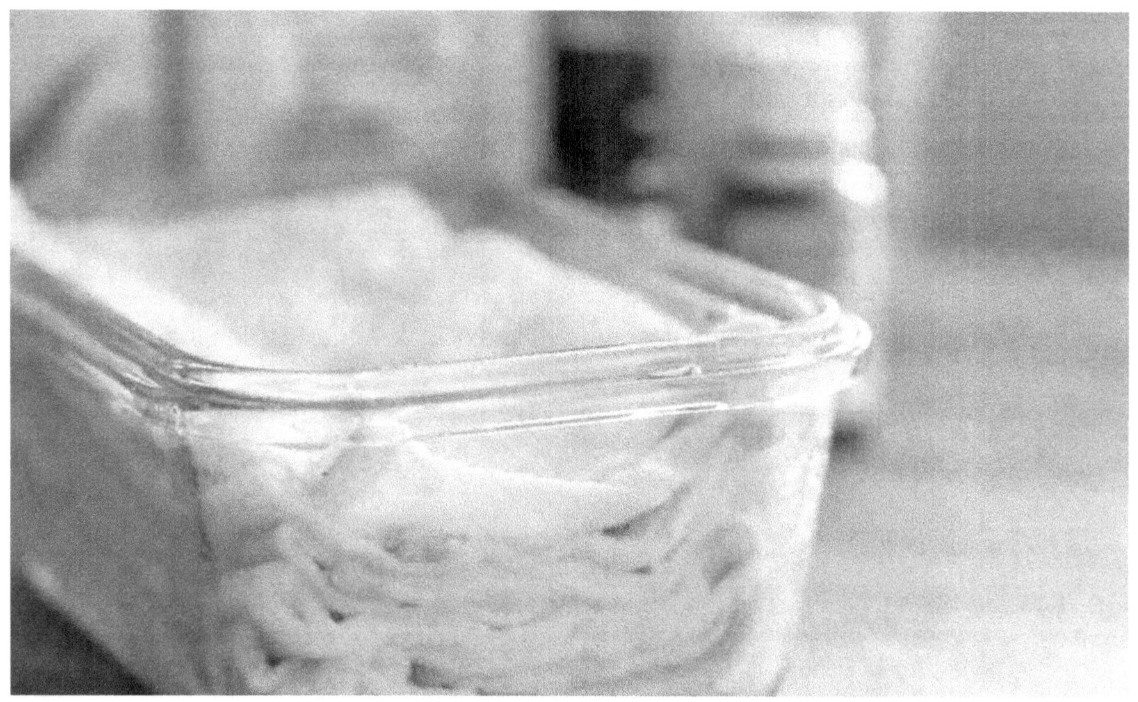

Try it with nutmeg! Makes 150-180 wipes

Ingredients:

- 1 ½ cup 70% isopropyl alcohol or 140 proof vodka
- 1 Tbsp coconut oil
- 5-8 drops cinnamon essential oil
- 20 drops lemon essential oil

Instructions:

Mix together alcohol or vodka with coconut oil, cinnamon & lemon essential oil.

Submerge towel or wipes in mixture.

Place in a container

Citrus Disinfecting Wipes

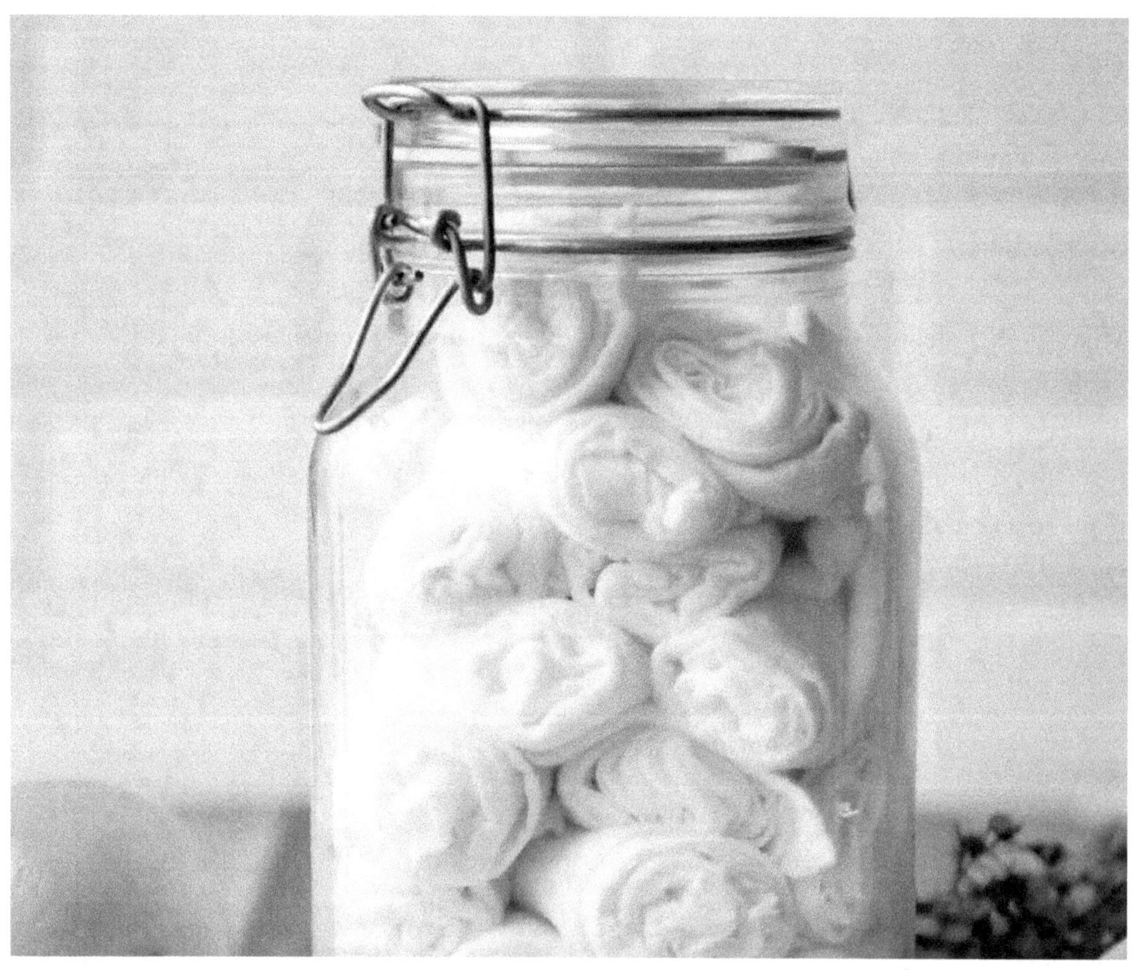

Great refreshing scent! Makes 150-180 wipes

Ingredients:

- 1 ½ cup 70% isopropyl alcohol or 140 proof vodka
- 1 Tbsp coconut oil
- 20 drops orange essential oil
- 5 drops lemon essential oil

Instructions:

Mix together alcohol or vodka with coconut oil, orange & lemon essential oil.

Submerge towel or wipes in mixture.

Place in a container.

Grapefruit & Lavender Disinfecting Spray

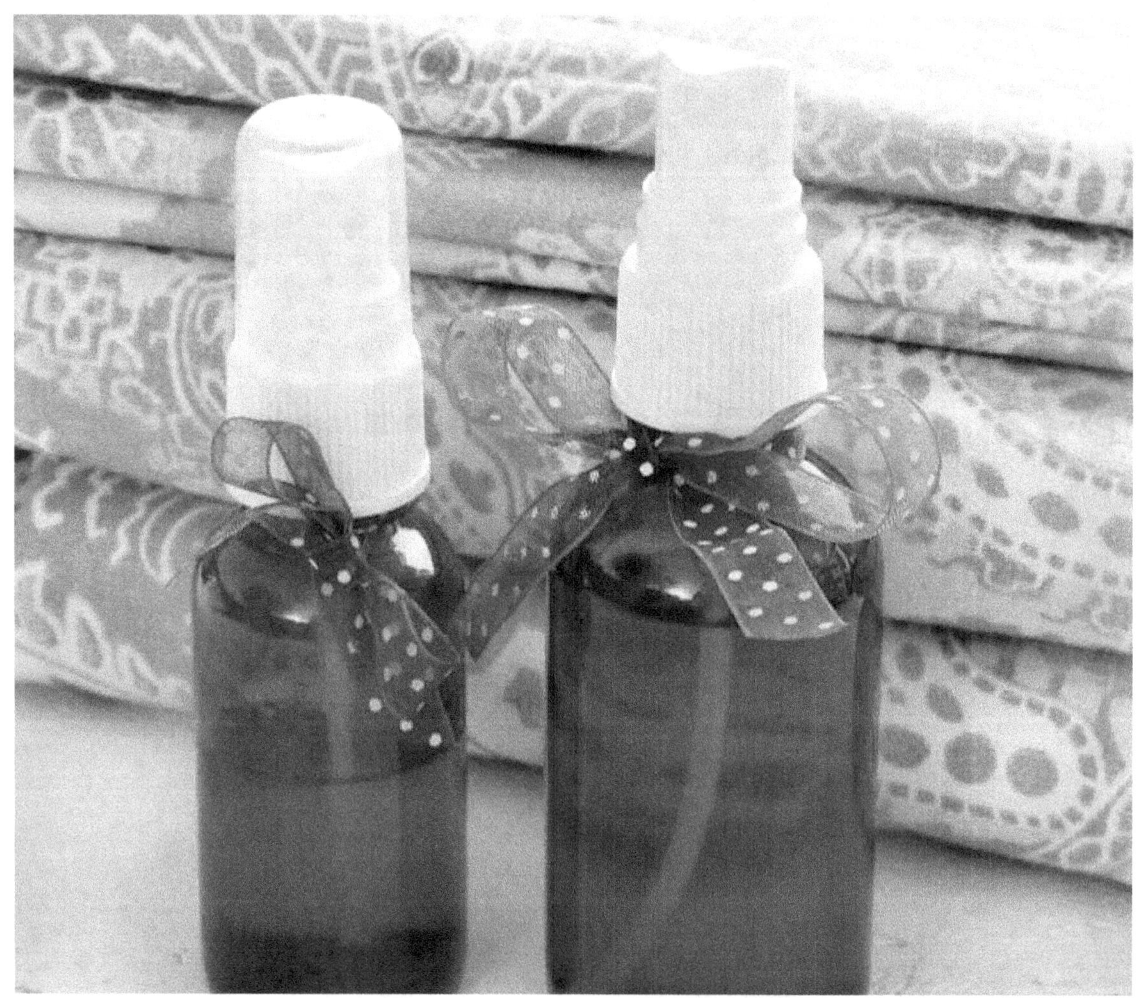

Let sit 10 minutes! Makes 8-24 oz.

Ingredients:

- 1 ½ cup 70% isopropyl alcohol or 140 proof vodka
- 1 Tbsp coconut oil
- 5-10 drops lavender essential oil
- 20-30 drops grapefruit essential oil

Instructions:

Mix together alcohol or vodka with coconut oil, lavender & lemon essential oil

Lemon Rose Disinfecting Wipes

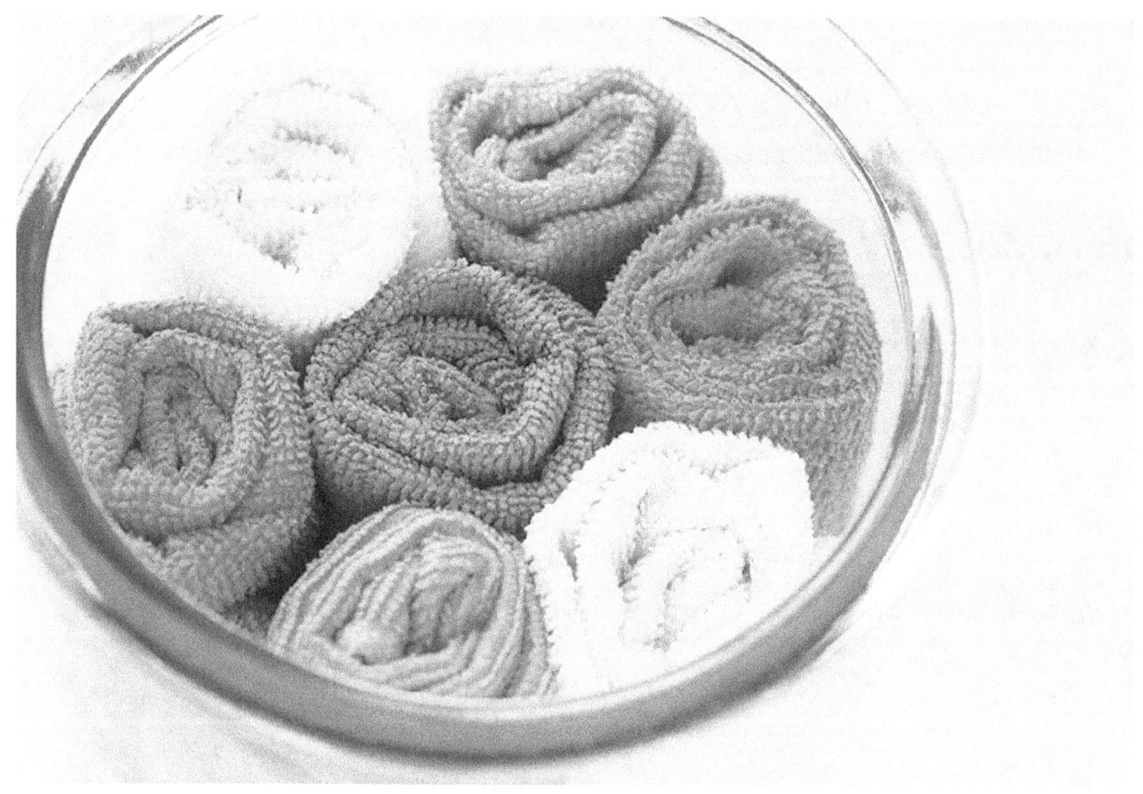

Great for spare bedrooms! Makes 150-180 wipes

Ingredients:

- 1 ½ cup 70% isopropyl alcohol or 140 proof vodka
- 1 Tbsp coconut oil
- 20 -25 drops rose essential oil
- 5-10 drops lemon essential oil

Instructions:

Mix together alcohol or vodka with coconut oil, rose & lemon essential oil.

Submerge towel or wipes in mixture.

Place in a container.

Eucalyptus Blu All-Purpose Cleaner Wipes with Vodka

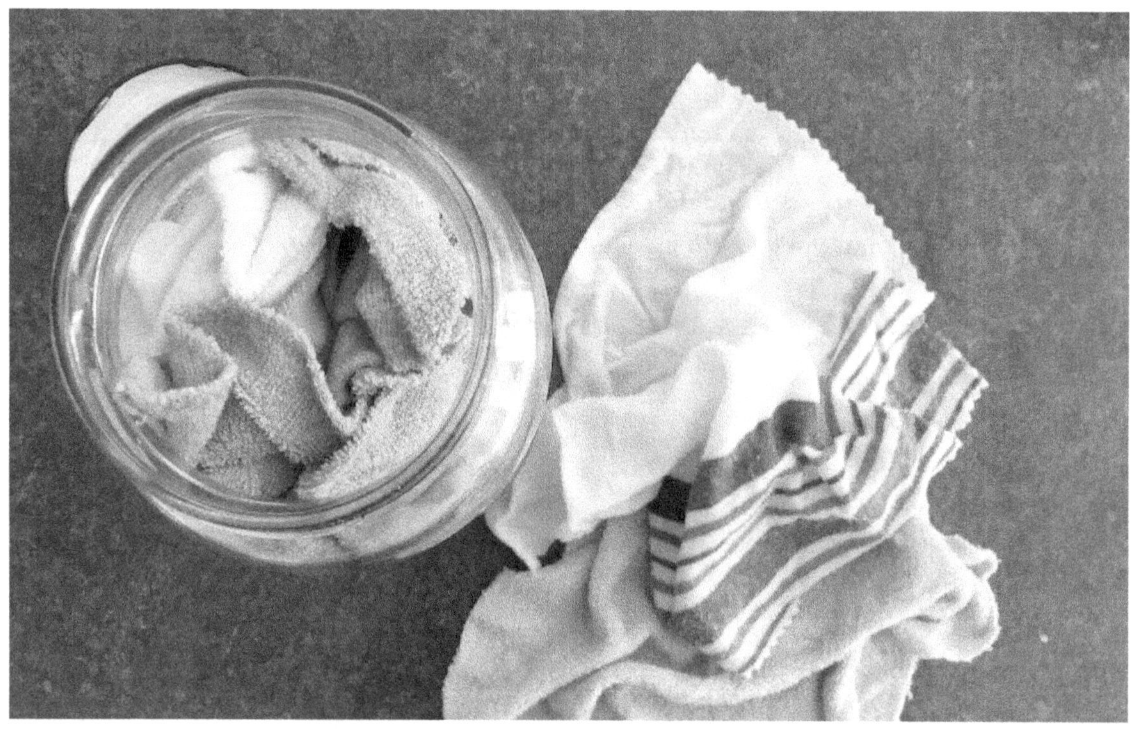

Great for garages, sheds, and man caves! Makes 150-180 wipes.

Ingredients:

- 2/3 cup vodka
- ¼ cup sterile hot water
- 1/3 of bottle with distilled vinegar
- 15 drops of thyme or tea tree oil
- 20-30 eucalyptus essential oil
- 2-4 drops of blue food coloring

Instructions:

Mix vodka, sterile water, vinegar, thyme or tea tree oil, eucalyptus & thyme essential oils, and food coloring together in bowl.

Submerge paper towels in mixture.

Place wipes in a container.

Will keep 2-4 weeks.

Heavy Duty Shop Wipes with Vodka

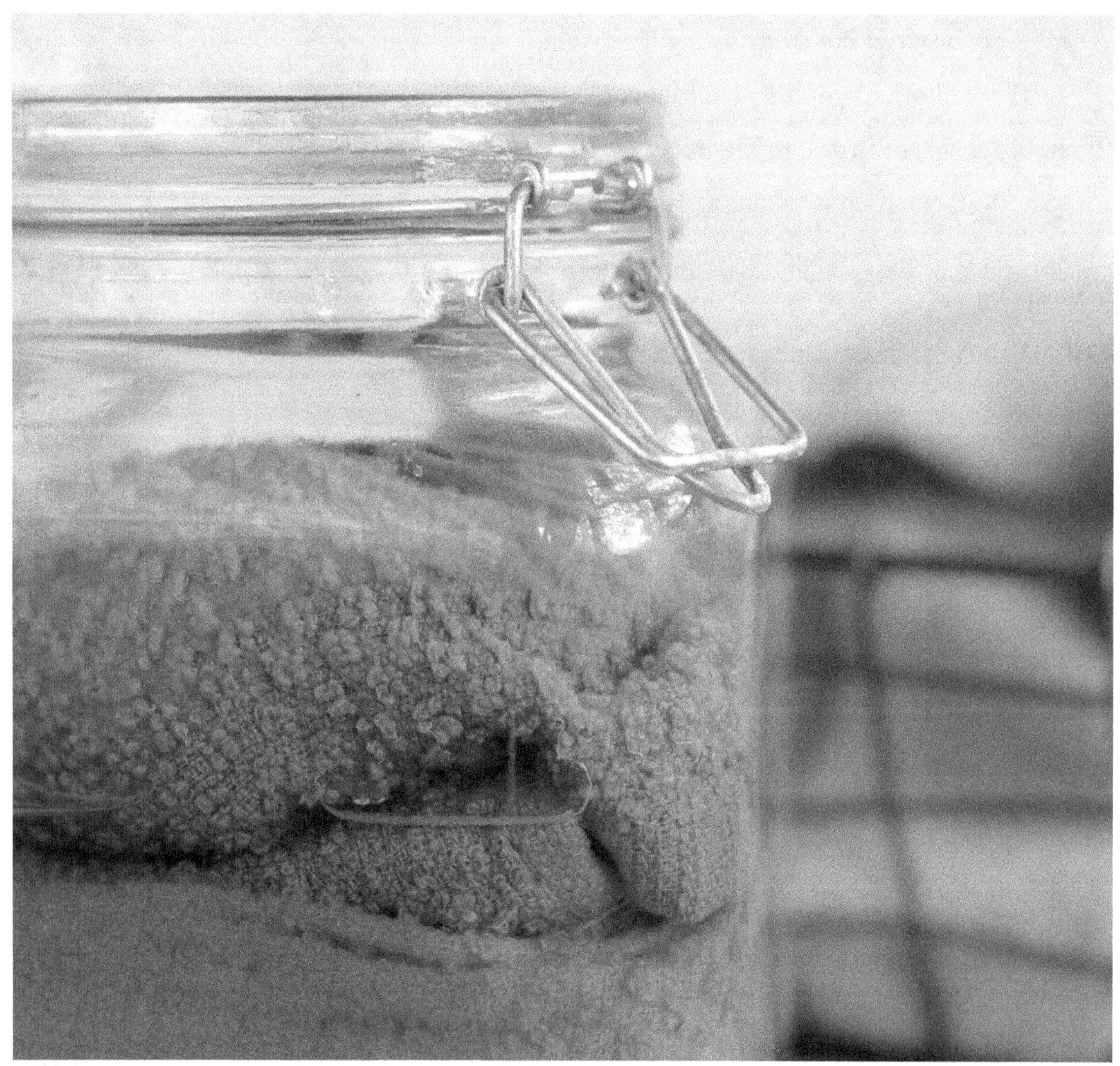

Power through germs! Makes 150-180 wipes.

Ingredients:

- 2/3 cup vodka
- ¼ cup sterile hot water
- 1/3 of bottle with distilled vinegar
- 5- 10 drops of thyme or tea tree oil
- 3-5 drops of cinnamon essential oil

Instructions:

Mix vodka, sterile water, vinegar, thyme or tea tree oil, and cinnamon essential oil together in bowl.

Submerge paper towels in mixture.

Place wipes in a container.

Will keep 2-4 weeks.

Black Rose Disinfecting Wipes

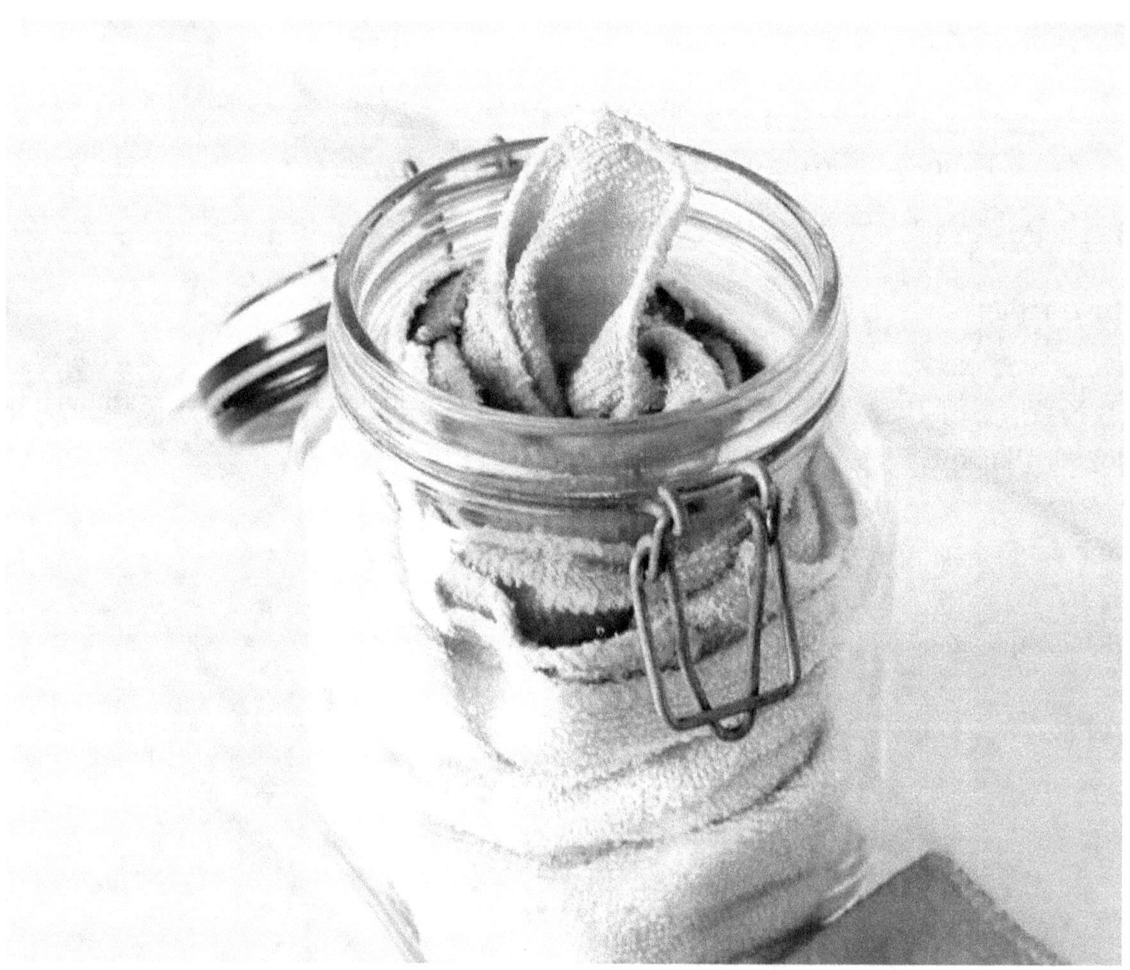

Great for teens! Makes 150-180 wipes.

Ingredients:

- 2/3 cup vodka
- ¼ cup sterile hot water
- 1/3 of bottle with distilled vinegar
- 3-5 drops of thyme or tea tree oil
- 20-30 rose essential oil
- 3-5 drops of black food coloring

Instructions:

Mix vodka, sterile water, vinegar, thyme or tea tree oil & rose essential oils, and food coloring together in bowl.

Submerge paper towels in mixture.

Place wipes in a container.

Will keep 2-4 weeks.

White Rose Wipes with Vodka

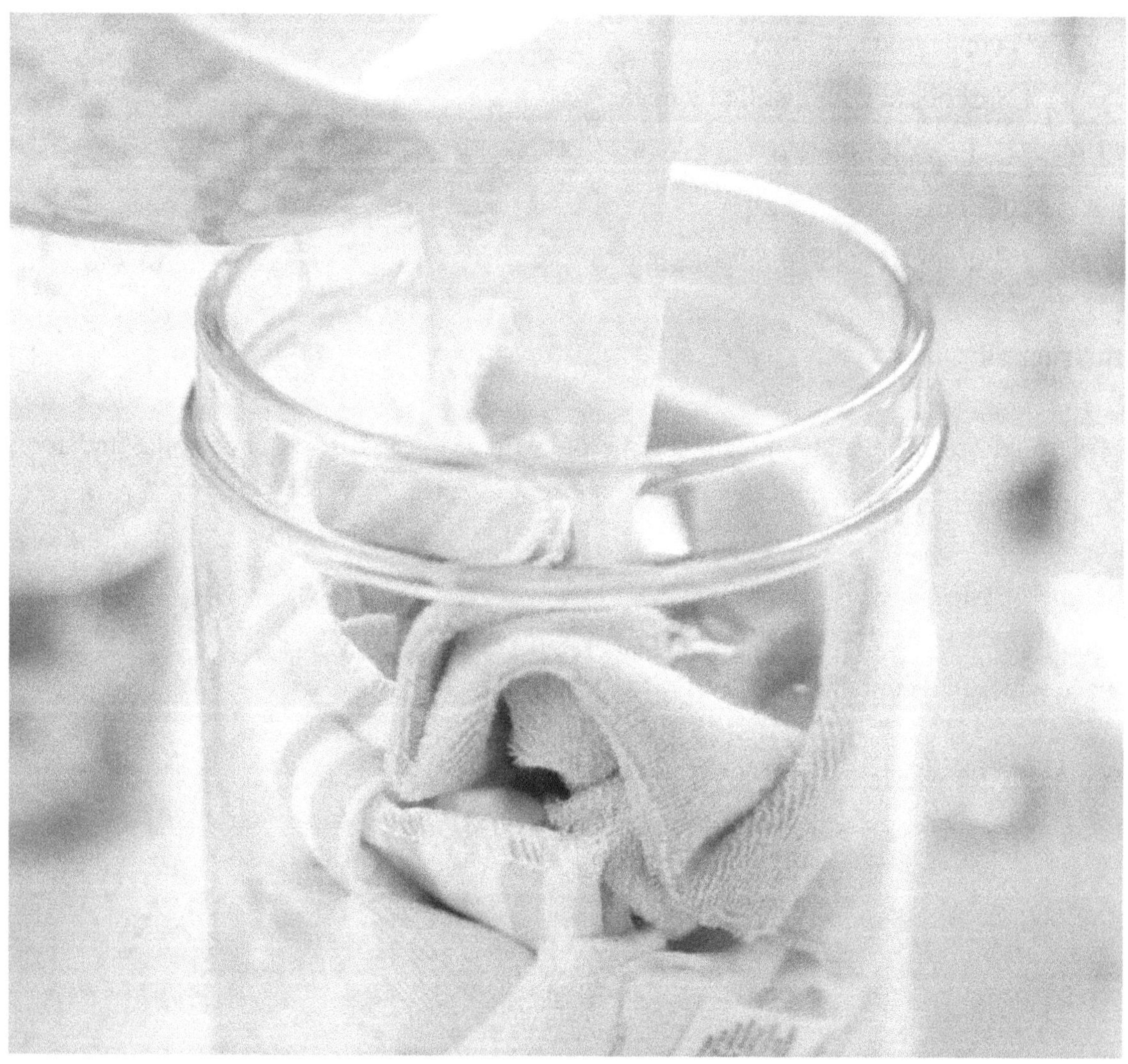

Make these red rose wipes! Makes 150-180 wipes.

Ingredients:

- 2/3 cup vodka
- ¼ cup sterile hot water
- 1/3 of bottle with distilled vinegar
- 3-5 drops of thyme or tea tree oil
- 30 rose essential oil

Instructions:

Mix vodka, sterile water, vinegar, thyme or tea tree oil & rose essential oil together in bowl.

Submerge paper towels in mixture.

Place wipes in a container.

Will keep 2-4 weeks.

Author's Afterthoughts

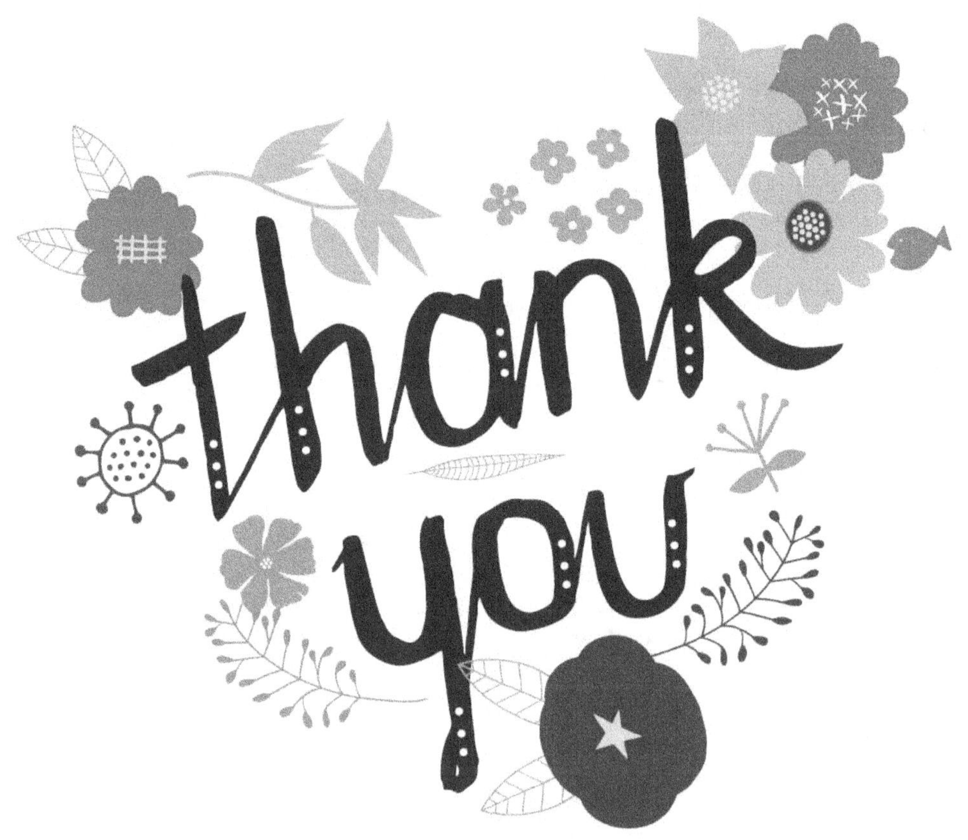

Thank you for reading my book. Your feedback is important to me. It would be greatly appreciated if you could please take a moment to REVIEW this book on Amazon so that we could make our next version better

Thanks!

Alice R. Groner